FAST FACTS

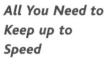

All You Need to Keep up to Speed

D0268785

Menopause

Second edition

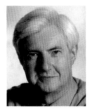

David H Barlow BSc MD FRCOG MRCP FMedSci

Executive Dean of Medicine and Professor of
  Reproductive Medicine
University of Glasgow
Glasgow, UK

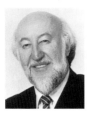

Barry G Wren AM MD MBBS MHPEd
            FRCOG FRANZCOG

Director (retired), Sydney Menopause Centre
Royal Hospital for Women
Sydney, Australia

Declaration of Independence

This book is as balanced and as practical as we can make it. Ideas for
improvement are always welcome: feedback@fastfacts.com

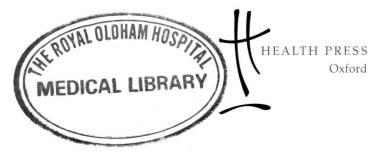

HEALTH PRESS
Oxford

Fast Facts – Menopause
First published 2000
Second edition August 2005

Text © 2005 David H Barlow, Barry G Wren
© 2005 in this edition Health Press Limited
Health Press Limited, Elizabeth House, Queen Street, Abingdon,
Oxford OX14 3LN, UK
Tel: +44 (0)1235 523233
Fax: +44 (0)1235 523238

Book orders can be placed by telephone or via the website.
For regional distributors or to order via the website, please go to:
www.fastfacts.com

For telephone orders, please call 01752 202301 (UK), +44 1752 202301 (Europe),
800 247 6553 (USA, toll free) or 419 281 1802 (Canada).

Fast Facts is a trademark of Health Press Limited.

The authors are grateful to Professor David F Archer of Eastern Virginia Medical
School, Norfolk, Virginia, USA, for his many contributions to the manuscript.

A CIP catalogue record for this title is available from the British Library.

ISBN 1-903734-38-X

Barlow DH (David H)
Fast Facts – Menopause/
David H Barlow, Barry G Wren

Medical illustrations by Dee McLean, London, UK.
Typesetting and page layout by Zed, Oxford, UK.
Printed by Fine Print (Services) Ltd, Oxford, UK.

Printed with vegetable inks on fully biodegradable and
recyclable paper manufactured from sustainable forests.

444   001
Low emissions
during production

Low   Sustainable
chlorine   forests

Glossary 4

Introduction 5

Stages, effects and implications 7

Vasomotor function 13

Osteoporosis 18

Urogenital changes 24

Neurological symptoms 29

Sexuality 34

Symptom management 37

Types of hormone therapy 46

Side effects of hormone therapy 55

Endometrial bleeding with hormone therapy 60

Risks of hormone therapy 63

Tibolone 89

Alternatives to hormone therapy 93

Useful resources 98

Appendix: Generic and proprietary names of estrogens 100

Index 103

Glossary

CEE: conjugated equine estrogen

CT: computed tomography

DXA: dual-energy X-ray absorption

EDRF: endothelial-derived relaxing factor

EPT: estrogen plus progestogen

FAI: free androgen index

FSH: follicle-stimulating hormone

HABITS: Hormone Replacement Therapy After Breast Cancer – Is It Safe?

HDL: high-density lipoprotein

HERS: Heart and Estrogen/Progestin Replacement Study

HT: hormone therapy (also called HRT)

HRT: hormone replacement therapy (also called HT)

LDL: low-density lipoprotein

MORE: Multiple Outcomes of Raloxifene Evaluation

NO: nitric oxide

SHBG: sex-hormone-binding globulin

SERM: selective estrogen-receptor modulator

SSRI: selective serotonin-reuptake inhibitor

STEAR: selective tissue estrogenic activity regulators

WHI: Women's Health Initiative

A note on terminology: We have used American spelling and terminology throughout this book. With respect to vasomotor symptoms, 'flashing' and 'hot flashes', as they are called in North America, are known in many parts of the English-speaking world as 'flushing' and 'hot flushes'.

Introduction

This concise handbook provides an overview of menopausal and postmenopausal health issues and their management. We have attempted to include a wide and relevant range of topics from our perspective as clinicians in women's postreproductive healthcare.

When discussing health topics, it is all too easy to focus on 'ill health' issues, as these tend to be the greatest concern for those seeking advice. It is therefore important to emphasize at the outset that, for a large number of women, the menopause is free of unpleasant symptoms, or relatively so. Many postmenopausal women will not experience osteoporosis, or the other problems discussed here, in later life and will lead active lives without using hormone therapy (HT). However, these diseases and other related conditions do have a major impact on the quality of life of some older women.

Common diseases in the elderly female population such as osteoporosis, cardiovascular disease, cerebrovascular disease and Alzheimer's disease pose a substantial financial burden on health resources, and knowledge about the effects, or lack of effects, of HT on these conditions has recently been considerably expanded. The potential impact of HT on both individual quality of life and overall healthcare costs is, therefore, an important issue beyond the usual boundaries of traditional 'women's healthcare'. The aims of this book are to increase understanding of the physiological and psychological effects of the menopause and, ultimately, to contribute to effective management.

Stages, effects and implications

Female reproductive maturity is characterized by monthly cycles of ovarian follicular development. The cycles govern a woman's circulating hormone levels and provide eggs for potential conception. The menopause is the inevitable consequence of the exhaustion of the supply of ovarian follicles, and can be regarded as a physiological form of ovarian failure.

Stages

Three terms are used to refer to the menopause, each with a slightly different meaning:
- perimenopause
- menopause
- climacteric.

Perimenopause. The transition into the perimenopause can be relatively sudden, but it usually lasts 3–5 years. In most women, there is a noticeable decline in the quality of ovarian function. This is indicated by a change in the pattern of menstruation from regular monthly cycles to erratic menstruation with reduced or increased menstrual intervals, or both. This change is usually due to the failure of regular ovulation.

While follicular development continues, significant estrogen production is maintained. However, a rise in the level of circulating follicle-stimulating hormone (FSH) can often be detected during the perimenopause, indicating a degree of failure in feedback from the ovarian hormones (Figure 1.1). Historically, it was assumed that this reflected impaired ovarian estrogen production, but research now suggests that the rise in FSH indicates a reduction in the secretion of the ovarian follicular peptide inhibin. Therefore, the perimenopause is characterized by impaired ovarian function and elevated blood FSH (Table 1.1); there may also be reduced estrogen levels overall.

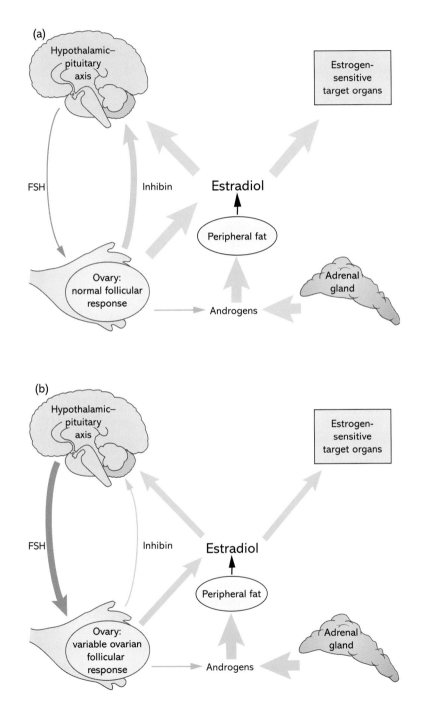

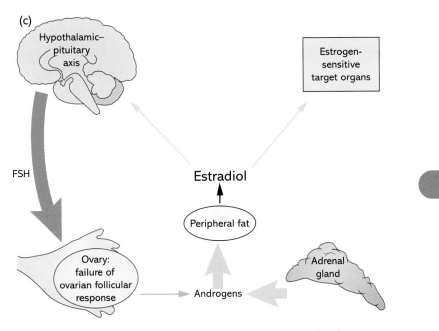

Figure 1.1 A summary of (a) premenopausal, (b) perimenopausal and (c) postmenopausal hormone production in women. The arrow size indicates the level of hormone secretion. FSH, follicle-stimulating hormone.

TABLE 1.1

Characteristics of the perimenopause

- Continuing but impaired ovarian function
- Increased blood levels of FSH
- Anovulatory cycles
- Erratic menstrual pattern
- Onset of menopausal symptoms
- Significantly reduced fertility
- Increased risk of fetal genetic abnormality

Menopause. Eventually, the ovarian 'cycles' produce insufficient estrogen to stimulate significant endometrial development and consequently menstruation ceases. This defines the menopause. It

9

usually occurs around the age of 50, but the exact timing cannot be certain until there is an interval – usually 6 months – with no withdrawal bleeds.

The climacteric is the transitional phase from mature reproductive function through the perimenopause to, essentially, no ovarian follicular function. Undoubtedly, this is a difficult time for many women because of the associated symptoms. However, population surveys show that the climacteric does not affect quality of life significantly in the majority of women.

The role of estrogen
In a reproductively mature woman, estrogen, produced primarily by the ovaries, has a number of important functions.
- Tissues in the breast, uterus, cervix, vagina and bladder are estrogen dependent.
- Bone mass is maintained by the influence of estrogen on bone turnover.
- Estrogen has a positive influence on many aspects of cardiovascular function, including maintenance of higher levels of high-density lipoprotein (HDL) cholesterol relative to low-density lipoprotein (LDL) cholesterol.
- The complex cycles that affect mood and sexual desire are influenced by estrogen.
- The deposition of toxic β-amyloid fragments within neurons that is an essential feature of Alzheimer's disease occurs more readily in the absence of estrogen.

Effects of hormone deficiency. Failure of the ovaries to produce estrogen has a detrimental effect on all of the systems in which the hormone has a role (Table 1.2). These are described in more detail in later chapters.

Hormone therapy
Hormone therapy (HT, sometimes called hormone replacement therapy, HRT) was initially instituted in the late 1930s. Its principal

TABLE 1.2

Symptoms of menopause

Affecting a majority

Vasomotor

- hot flashes
- night sweats (severe in a minority)

Affecting a minority

Psychological

- lack of confidence
- poor memory
- lack of concentration
- depressed mood
- anxiety

General

- tiredness
- headaches
- insomnia

Sexual

- lack of libido

Vaginal

- discomfort
- dyspareunia
- burning or itching

Urinary tract symptoms

- frequency
- recurrent urinary tract infection
- urgency
- stress incontinence

aim is to maintain or restore quality of life for women who experience symptoms or who wish to brake the deleterious age-related changes that accelerate in the absence of appropriate sex hormones.

When HT was initially developed, estrogen was administered in a continuous, unopposed manner. Within two decades, however, this was found to be associated with a significant increase in the incidence of uterine cancer. Consequently, a progestogen was added to the regimen for 7–14 days of the cycle to prevent an abnormal response in endometrial cells. This cyclical progestogen regimen induced a withdrawal bleed, with increased mastalgia and mood changes. Attempts to overcome these problems led to the introduction of many different preparations and regimens (see Chapter 8). Today, the most frequently prescribed HT regimens are sequential estrogen and progestogen preparations, which are suitable for perimenopausal or postmenopausal women, and continuous combined estrogen and progestogen preparations, which are suitable for postmenopausal women. For women who have had a hysterectomy the standard approach to HT is to use estrogen without progestogen, usually referred to as estrogen-only HT.

The recent publication of the Women's Health Initiative (WHI) study, the first large, long-term randomized controlled trial of HT use in 'healthy' postmenopausal women, has brought about a reappraisal of the effects of HT, particularly in relation to cardiovascular disease (see Table 11.2, page 70).

Key points – stages, effects and implications

- The menopausal transition involves the failure of ovarian cyclical activity, which is the major source of estrogen in women before the menopause.
- The transition may be associated with menstrual irregularity or menopausal symptoms; however, many women experience no problems.
- The postmenopausal phase is characterized by an absence of menstrual periods, high blood levels of follicle-stimulating hormone and low blood estrogen levels.
- In the postmenopausal decades, women who are deficient in estrogen appear to have an accelerated onset of osteoporosis, cardiovascular and cerebrovascular disease and Alzheimer's disease.
- Because of recent epidemiological studies suggesting an adverse outcome when using hormone therapy, there is considerable controversy over the management of women experiencing symptoms.

The hot flashes (known as 'hot flushes' outside North America) and night sweats commonly associated with menopause are a consequence of vasomotor dysfunction. The frequency and intensity of the symptoms vary between women, and over time for an individual woman. Such vasomotor events are part of a normal physiological response to fever, but during menopausal flashes the body's core temperature is not elevated. These symptoms often commence in the perimenopausal phase, but are also common in the postmenopausal phase. Up to 80% of peri- and postmenopausal women experience vasomotor symptoms, but only half of these women are sufficiently affected to consider therapy.

Causes

The causes of vasomotor symptoms are not clear. It is likely that a fall in estrogen, whether transient or sustained, affects central neurotransmitter activity, including activity at the thermoregulatory center in the hypothalamus. Estradiol has been shown to modulate neuronal activity in several neurotransmitter systems, including the serotonin, norepinephrine and endogenous opiate pathways.

In general, the mechanisms correlate with the menopausal decline in estrogen levels, which eventually stabilize in the postmenopausal years. Women experiencing intermittent low levels of estrogen during the perimenopause often experience flashes even though they have adequate levels of estrogen most of the time. Despite these correlations, studies of endocrine parameters have not established direct associations between flashes and specific hormone levels.

The physiological changes that occur during flashes have been defined by biophysical studies. The woman is aware of a

13

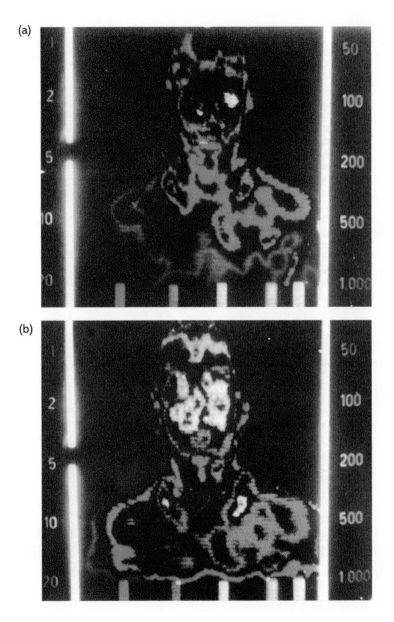

Figure 2.1 Thermograms showing the distribution of heat in a menopausal woman (a) before and (b) during a hot flash. The temperature increase is indicated in steps of 1 °C from red to green to white. Adapted from Sturdee DW et al. *Maturitas* 1979;1:201–5.

sensation of heat, lasting 4–5 minutes, that affects the upper body primarily, and the face and neck in particular (Figure 2.1). The sensation is due to rapid vasodilation of the skin blood vessels, which is associated with an increase in heart rate and a reduction in skin resistance. The skin temperature rises several degrees centigrade and the core temperature falls slightly. Sweats have similar features, but are common at night and tend to be more prolonged. Some women also experience formication (a sensation like ants crawling on the skin), while others feel faint or dizzy in association with flashes or sweats.

Peripheral vasodilation principally reflects sympathetic vasomotor tone. There is a rapid fluctuation between increased and decreased sympathetic tone, inducing vasoconstriction and vasodilation, respectively. Studies have indicated that women who experience flashes have different sympathetic vasomotor control from those who experience few symptoms, but physiological insights into flashes have not led to specific therapies. Treatment is simply determined according to the symptoms and to the extent to which the woman wishes for relief from the symptoms.

Key points – vasomotor function

- Hot flashes affect most perimenopausal or postmenopausal women at some time.
- Surgical menopause after bilateral oophorectomy is especially likely to be associated with distressing hot flashes.
- For most women, hot flashes subside over several years, but for some the symptoms persist till death, being triggered by simple events such as a cup of tea or mild exertion.
- Hot flashes or night sweats can be distressing and are a common reason that women use hormone therapy.
- Some women experience a sensation like ants crawling on their skin, while others feel faint or dizzy in association with flashes or sweats.

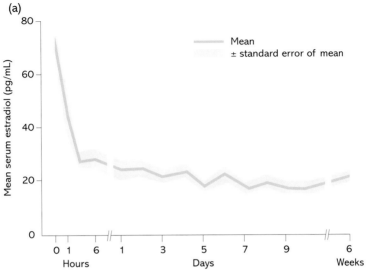

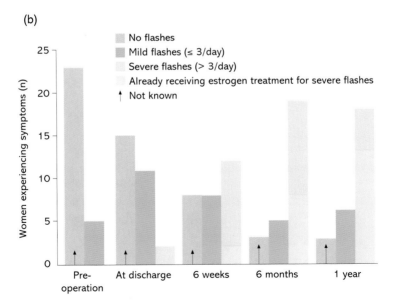

Figure 2.2 The effect of premenopausal bilateral oophorectomy on (a) serum estradiol and (b) the development of hot flashes (Barlow DH, Blair-Bell Memorial Lecture, Royal College of Obstetricians and Gynaecologists, 1985).

Flashes following surgical menopause can be a particular problem. Surgical removal of the ovaries (bilateral oophorectomy) causes a dramatic drop in levels of circulating estradiol within hours. This sudden transition is associated with a particularly high risk of flashes (Figure 2.2). This risk is the same for women close to the menopause and those who had full reproductive function before having surgery. A follow-up study has shown that most women undergoing surgical menopause develop particularly distressing flashes, but that the full extent of the problem is often not established at the time of discharge from hospital or even at follow-up 6 weeks later.

Key references

Brockie JA, Barlow DH, Rees MC. Menopausal flush symptomatology and sustained reflex vasoconstriction. *Hum Reprod* 1991;6:472–4.

Oldenhave A, Jaszmann LJ, Haspels AA, Everaerd WT. Impact of climacteric on well-being. A survey based on 5213 women 39 to 60 years old. *Am J Obstet Gynecol* 1993;168: 772–80.

Sturdee DW, Wilson KA, Pipili E, Crocker AD. Physiological aspects of menopausal hot flush. *BMJ* 1978;2: 79–80.

Osteoporosis is a disease of low bone mass with accompanying architectural impairment of bone, which leads to an increased risk of fracture. In postmenopausal women, an increased risk of osteoporosis is a consequence of the changes in calcium metabolism that result from the fall in level of circulating estrogen.

Osteoporosis places the largest financial burden on healthcare resources of the postmenopausal problems. It is a major cause of disability in later life, and is associated with considerable cost to the NHS in the UK, currently estimated to be approximately £2 billion per annum. In the USA, the National Osteoporosis Foundation estimates the direct costs of osteoporosis at $17 billion; in Australia the direct inpatient costs are estimated to be A$1.5 billion annually, while indirect costs to the total community are a further A$1 billion.

The treatment of osteoporosis is described in Chapter 7.

Bone

Bone mass and turnover are mediated by the activity of bone-resorbing osteoclasts and bone-forming osteoblasts so that bone modeling and remodeling is a continual process throughout life. Finely tuned control mechanisms normally balance the opposing functions in adults so that overall bone mass remains relatively static, or declines only slowly with advancing age. Where physical demands change, there can be adjustment of the bone mass to match; for example, an increase in the bone mass of the serving arm in tennis players, or a reduction in bone mass during the weightlessness of space flight. At menopause, estrogen deficiency increases the rate of bone resorption. Although the rate at which bone is formed subsequently rises to counterbalance this, the increase is not sufficient to maintain overall bone mass (Figure 3.1). This loss of bone mass is not seen in men of the same age.

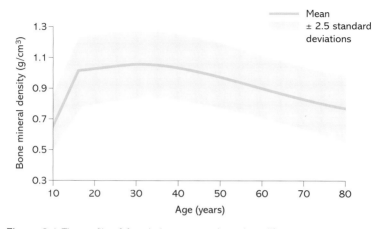

Figure 3.1 The profile of female bone mass throughout life.

A woman's peak bone mass is a result of her genetic potential, diet, exercise pattern and estrogen status during the years of reproductive maturity. From the time of the menopause, these factors are undermined by the sustained fall in estrogen. The most rapid loss occurs in the early postmenopausal years, but excess bone resorption tends to continue long term.

Bone mass assessment. Bone mass is measured by densitometry, usually by dual-energy X-ray densitometry (DXA or DEXA; see below). The resulting measurement is reported in relation to a curve of distribution of bone density measurements, either the curve for people of the same age and gender as the person being tested (the Z score) or the curve for young adults of the same gender (the T score) (Figure 3.2). The score is expressed in statistical terms as units of standard deviation (SD). The Z score is relative, indicating how an individual is placed for age, but for a more absolute diagnostic standard the T score is used. Osteoporosis is defined as a T score 2.5 SDs or more below the young adult mean (see Figure 3.2). There is good evidence that the fracture risk doubles for a reduction of 1 SD in T score. Currently an international project is developing methods that combine bone density

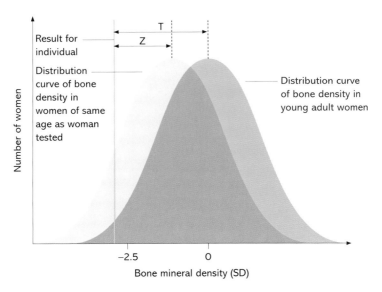

Figure 3.2 A graphical representation of the T and Z scores. The woman tested (green line) is sufficiently postmenopausal for the mean to be shifted downwards (blue curve), but her Z score is below the mean for her age. The T score is below −2.5 standard deviations, and therefore she has osteoporosis.

measurements, age and other risk factors to permit calculation of an individual's absolute fracture risk estimate. This would be a major advance in the field.

Bone densitometry. Bone density can be determined by a number of methods, including single- and dual-photon absorptiometry, computed tomography (CT) and ultrasound. The best-validated method at present is DXA. Access to densitometry technology varies widely, and there is much discussion concerning the appropriate use of these techniques.

The current gold standard for diagnosing osteoporosis is spinal and total hip DXA. This may also be useful in predicting fracture risk, since a 1 SD reduction in T score is approximately equivalent to a doubling of fracture risk at the same site. DXA at one site is less good at predicting fracture risk at other sites, although it is still useful for this purpose. The role of DXA in monitoring osteoporosis is undergoing reappraisal. Certainly, monitoring intervals should not be closer than 2 years because of the limited sensitivity of the method. Furthermore, it is now argued that the use of DXA in the monitoring of therapy is not cost-effective, since a large majority of women on validated therapies do respond. It is likely that in future, when response to therapy is to be assessed, bone biochemical markers will be used.

Peripheral DXA is attracting attention as a less expensive option than spine and hip DXA. However, such peripheral measurements are of less value in diagnosing osteoporosis and predicting fracture risk at the major fracture sites.

Heel ultrasound assessment undoubtedly provides valuable information and is less expensive than DXA. However, its value in diagnosing osteoporosis and predicting fracture risk has yet to be fully validated. Heel ultrasound is a better predictor of risk of fracture than patient history, and it may therefore prove to be a more useful initial screening tool than family history in selecting women suitable for spine and hip DXA assessment.

Fractures

The most common and significant sites of fracture are the spine, hip and wrist (Table 3.1). From their late fifties onwards, women are at

---

Key points – osteoporosis

- The bone mass achieved in adults is the result of multiple influences including genetic factors, physical activity and diet, particularly calcium intake.
- Bone mass is maintained by the balance of bone-cell activity, and after the menopause this balance changes, so that bone mass declines.
- Osteoporosis is a potentially debilitating condition that occurs most commonly in postmenopausal women as a result of the decline in bone mass that follows the menopause.
- Postmenopausal fracture is usually the consequence of osteo-porosis and most commonly occurs at the spine, wrist and hip.

TABLE 3.1

Common osteoporotic fractures

Vertebral fracture

Not necessarily associated with trauma

Can cause deformity of spine and significant disability

Occurs mainly from the age of 60 years onwards

Causes individual disability, but does not have significant economic implications for health providers

No hospitalization necessary so health statistics are incomplete

Hip fracture

Associated with falls

Occurs mainly from the age of 70 years onwards

Significant 1-year mortality

Accurate statistics available as all cases require hospitalization

The major component of the burden of osteoporosis for health services

Subsequent loss of independence in the elderly is common

Wrist (Colles') fracture

Associated with falls

Occurs at any age, but mainly from the age of 60 years onwards

Variable continuing disability

Accurate statistics available as all cases have hospital involvement

particular risk of vertebral fractures, which result in deformity and discomfort. Such fractures often occur silently and have not been thought to be a financial burden to health-service providers; however, recent evidence from Sweden suggests that the costs may be greatly underestimated. In contrast, hip fractures are known to be a major drain on health-service resources, as they inevitably require hospitalization and surgery. Hip fractures are most common in women over 70 years of age and in association with falls – they occur twice as often in women as in men. Following such a fracture, some individuals are no longer able to lead an independent life.

Key references

Cauley JA, Seeley DG, Ensrud K et al. Estrogen therapy and fractures in older women. Study of Osteoporotic Fractures Research Group. *Ann Intern Med* 1995;122: 9–16.

Marshall D, Johnell O, Wedel H. Meta-analysis of how well measures of bone mineral density predict occurrences of osteoporotic fractures. *BMJ* 1996;312:1254–9.

Urogenital tissues are estrogen sensitive and, following the menopause, they undergo changes that are often referred to as urogenital atrophy. The characteristic features include:

- epithelial thinning
- reduced vascularity
- decreased muscle bulk
- increased fat deposition.

At a cellular level, there is fatty infiltration, elastic tissue degeneration and loss of cell definition (Table 4.1). The tissues shrink and vaginal secretions tend to reduce with time.

The reduction in vaginal cellular glycogen is associated with a lower level of *Lactobacillus* colonization. There is a subsequent decrease in the amount of lactic acid produced by the *Lactobacilli*, which causes the vaginal pH to become relatively neutral (6–8) instead of acidic (4–5).

Possible treatments for the symptoms of urogenital atrophy are discussed in Chapter 7.

Symptoms

Vaginal irritation, dryness, dyspareunia and itching are all associated with urogenital atrophy. The loss of elasticity and decreased thickness of the epithelium cause the vagina to be more easily traumatized, and can result in vaginal bleeding. Symptoms are similar to those of recurrent urinary tract infection, urinary frequency or urge incontinence. All postmenopausal women not taking HT will have a relative estrogen deficiency, so a large proportion may experience these symptoms. Despite this, surveys of healthy postmenopausal women suggest that the majority are not significantly distressed by urogenital symptoms. However, those women who would like to remain sexually active should be differentiated from those who no longer have a desire to indulge in sexual activity; a number of women cease intercourse because it becomes too painful.

TABLE 4.1

Changes in the urinary tract and vagina associated with urogenital atrophy

Urinary tract

Trigonal urethral epithelial thinning

Decreased urethral plexus flow

Decreased connective tissue volume and elasticity

Striated muscle atrophy

Decreased periurethral α-adrenergic receptors

Loss of bladder glycosaminoglycans leading to bacterial invasion and urinary tract infection

Vaginal

Epithelium less cellular

Reduced elasticity and distensibility, dyspareunia

Easily traumatized, resulting in postmenopausal bleeding

Loss of cellular glycogen

Decreased lactic acid results in pH changing from 4/5 to 6–8; more neutral environment increases susceptibility to pathogenic/enteric invasion

Decreased blood flow

Prevalence. A representative population survey of older women in the UK showed that only about 10% were affected by any single symptom (Table 4.2). However, urogenital aging involves several possible symptoms; almost half the women (49%) had experienced urogenital symptoms at some time and approximately one-third (31%) had had symptoms during the 2 years prior to the survey. It is important that women receive information about this aspect of postmenopausal health, as many are reluctant to discuss urogenital problems with healthcare professionals. In a recent survey, women in six European countries showed similar patterns of response to these problems (Table 4.3). Older women should be made to feel comfortable discussing what they may regard as an embarrassing issue.

TABLE 4.2

Prevalence of symptoms of urogenital aging reported by women in the UK

| | Age group (years) | | | |
	55–64 (n = 706)	65–74 (n = 678)	75–84 (n = 517)	85+ (n = 109)
Vaginal itching	10%	11%	12%	13%
Dryness	11%	7%	7%	2%
Dyspareunia	3%	1%	0.4%	0
Urgency/dysuria/ frequency	14%	14%	18%	18%
Incontinence	7%	7%	13%	14%

Data from Barlow DH et al. *Br J Obstet Gynaecol* 1996;104:87–91.

Assessment

A vulvar and vaginal examination is necessary to assess urogenital atrophy. However, there is not always a close correlation between an atrophic appearance and the presence of symptoms. Many

TABLE 4.3

A survey of the attitude of 3000 European women to symptoms of urogenital atrophy

	Embarrassed to see doctor	Medical help sought	No help sought
Denmark	7%	53%	35%
France	16%	68%	26%
Germany	11%	44%	41%
Italy	12%	67%	20%
Netherlands	9%	58%	36%
UK	22%	53%	35%

Data from Barlow DH et al. *Maturitas* 1997;27:239–47.

women with clinically apparent atrophic tissues remain asymptomatic. The clinical picture includes pallor of thin-looking vaginal skin, in which the extent of rugae is reduced. Objective assessment can include a vaginal smear. For urogenital atrophy, this will show a failure of epithelial maturation with a marked reduction in the proportion of superficial epithelial cells and a relative excess of parabasal epithelial cells. This pattern is reflected in indices such as the maturation index (percentage of superficial cells).

In cases of incontinence, the options for objective assessment are pelvic examination, urine culture and, possibly, urodynamic investigation. It is important to establish whether there is any clinical evidence of uterine or vaginal prolapse.

Diagnosis

If symptoms are suggestive of urinary tract infection, such as frequency, urgency or dysuria, urine culture is important. If culture studies fail to demonstrate infection, the symptoms are likely to be a manifestation of urogenital atrophy.

Key points – urogenital changes

- After the menopause, low estrogen levels are associated with atrophic changes in the estrogen-sensitive pelvic tissues.
- These atrophic changes may cause vaginal or bladder symptoms, which may continue long term.
- The atrophic changes are very common but only a minority of postmenopausal women are distressed by the symptoms.
- Findings on clinical examination may correlate poorly with symptoms.
- If symptoms suggestive of urinary tract infection are associated with negative urine culture, urogenital atrophy is a likely cause.

Key references

Barlow DH, Cardozo LD, Francis RM et al. Urogenital ageing and its effect on sexual health in older British women. *Br J Obstet Gynaecol* 1997;104:87–91.

Barlow DH, Samsioe G, van Geelen JM. A study of European women's experience of the problems of urogenital ageing and its management. *Maturitas* 1997; 27:239–47.

Bidmead J, Cardozo LD. Pelvic floor changes in the older woman. *Br J Urol* 1998;82(suppl 1):18–25.

Cardozo LD, Bachmann G, McClish D et al. Meta-analysis of estrogen therapy in the management of urogenital atrophy in postmenopausal women: second report of the Hormones and Urogenital Therapy Committee. *Obstet Gynecol* 1998;92:722–7.

Stamm WE, Raz R. Factors contributing to susceptibility of postmenopausal women to recurrent urinary tract infections. *Clin Infect Dis* 1999;28:723–5.

Before publication of the results of the WHI trial (see Table 11.2, page 70), a substantial body of mechanistic and observational study evidence suggested a beneficial role for estrogen. The WHI trial, in an older postmenopausal group of women (over 65 years), did not find benefit and suggested an increase in the risk of dementia in those who used estrogen. Consequently, the effect of HT on the brain has become highly controversial.

Survey evidence suggests that some symptoms of psychological dysfunction peak at the menopausal transition (Figure 5.1). However, there is a lack of evidence that these symptoms are a direct result of estrogen deficiency. Some researchers attribute these symptoms to a combination of chronic insomnia resulting from night sweats, other life events and a predisposition to psychological problems in some women.

Estrogen and neurological function

Receptors for estrogen, progesterone and testosterone are found in a number of specific centers within the brain. It is therefore likely that menopause will result in malfunction of some important neurological activities. As well as the loss of functional memory, cells may be permanently damaged, leading ultimately to dementia. It has been estimated that approximately 15–20% of women over 75 suffer from some form of mental deterioration, the most common being Alzheimer's disease; another estimate, based on the WHI study, suggests that about 33% of women and only 20% of men over the age of 65 years experience dementia. The difference is thought to be related to the menopause.

Mechanisms. Several mechanisms have been proposed to explain how estrogen deficiency might affect neurological function. It is possible that each one, outlined below, contributes to the degenerative processes in neurons.

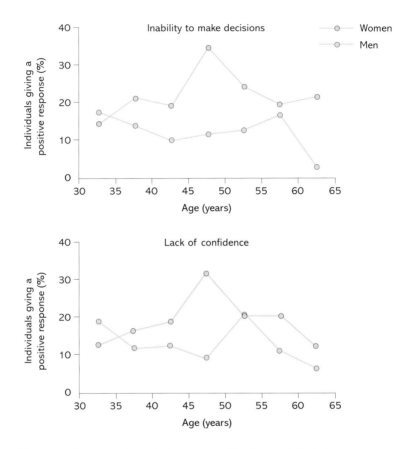

Figure 5.1 In a general population survey, subjective psychological symptoms, such as (a) experiencing difficulty in making decisions and (b) a loss of confidence, peak in women around the time of the menopause. Adapted from Bungay GT et al. *BMJ* 1980;281:181–3.

- Cerebral blood flow and vasodilation are reduced in all peripheral vessels.
- There is an increased risk of atherosclerosis and thrombosis in cerebral vessels (atherosclerotic microvascular thrombosis normally accounts for 20% of all dementia).
- Estrogen promotes in-vitro growth of neurons and appears to play a major role in neurological repair processes via nerve growth factors. These effects are reduced after the menopause.

- Synaptic density and plasticity decrease with reduced levels of estrogen.
- Estrogen deficiency results in decreased production of neurotransmitters, such as acetylcholine and serotonin, and reduced neuronal activity.
- The production of brain-derived neurotrophic factors and nerve growth factors, which are responsible for delaying the age-related degeneration of brain cells, is decreased.
- The process by which toxic β-amyloid fragments are deposited within neurons occurs more readily in the absence of estrogen. This deposition is an essential feature of Alzheimer's disease.
- Glucose metabolism within the hippocampus is maintained within normal levels in the presence of estrogen. Postmenopausal women deprived of estrogen experience severe glycopenia, which results in accelerated neuronal damage.

Symptoms

Many menopausal women complain of symptoms suggestive of a deterioration in memory and neurological function. Subjective descriptions of confusion, agitation, nervousness, forgetfulness, feeling 'woolly-headed', depression, lack of self-confidence and self-esteem, and loss of drive and energy are common. These symptoms are present in 30–50% of women, and are often misdiagnosed or inappropriately treated.

Alzheimer's disease has been found in observational studies to develop in 5% of women over 75 who have taken estrogen from the time of the menopause compared with more than 16% of those who have never used estrogen. When the signs of dementia have become apparent, it is clearly too late to treat most sufferers.

Memory. In the brain, estrogen receptors exist in the cerebral cortex, hypothalamus and pituitary gland. There is a large accumulation of sex-steroid receptors in the limbic area, which is responsible for memory as well as the affective sensations. Estrogen is involved in the processes of prenatal growth of dendrites, synaptic connection and neuronal differentiation in the brain that influence female verbal abilities, perceptual speed and fine motor skills. Following menopause, a number of these skills begin to deteriorate and a noticeable diminution of neurological function occurs.

Depression. Women who suffer from symptoms of estrogen deficiency may feel terrible, with associated reactive depression.

Key points – neurological symptoms

- Dementia is more common in older women than in men.
- Psychological dysfunction, mood changes, forgetfulness, confusion and loss of confidence are common in perimenopausal women.
- Brain-cell receptors for estrogen, progesterone and testosterone have been identified in specific cells in different regions of the brain.
- Estrogen stimulates neuritic growth factors.
- β-amyloid deposition is reduced in women who continue estrogen use from the time of the menopause.
- In observational studies, estrogen use from the time of the menopause is associated with decreased evidence of dementia.
- Estrogen use after the age of 65 failed to reduce the risk of Alzheimer's disease recorded in the Women's Health Initiative trial, and may even increase the risk of dementia.
- Estrogen use after the onset of Alzheimer's disease has no beneficial effect.

Key references

Espeland MA, Rapp SR, Shumaker SA et al. Women's Health Initiative Memory Study. Conjugated equine estrogens and global cognitive function in postmenopausal women. *JAMA* 2004;291:2959–68.

McEwen BS. Clinical Review 108: The molecular and neuroanatomical basis for estrogen effects in the central nervous system. *J Clin Endocrinol Metab* 1999;84:1790–7.

Shumaker SA, Legault C, Kuller L et al. Women's Health Initiative Memory Study. Conjugated equine estrogens and incidence of probable dementia and mild cognitive impairment in postmenopausal women. *JAMA* 2004;291:2947–58.

Shumaker SA, Legault C, Rapp SR et al. Women's Health Initiative Memory Study. Estrogen plus progestin and the incidence of dementia and mild cognitive impairment in postmenopausal women: the Women's Health Initiative Memory Study: a randomized controlled trial. *JAMA* 2003;289:2651–2662.

Tang MY, Jacobs D, Stern Y et al. Effect of oestrogen during menopause on risk and age of onset of Alzheimer's Disease. *Lancet* 1996;348:429–32.

Xu H, Gouras GK, Greenfield JP et al. Estrogen reduces neuronal generation of Alzheimer beta-amyloid peptides. *Nat Med* 1998; 4:447–51.

Yaffe K. Hormone therapy and the brain: deja vu all over again? *JAMA* 2003;289:2717–18.

Sexuality and libido are closely associated with sexual response in both men and women. It is therefore not unusual for reduced sexual desire or response to be related to decreased levels of sex hormones. Generally, a loss of libido can be ascribed to one of the three main areas described below, although all components may be involved to a certain degree:

- self-respect and self-image
- partner
- somatic sexual regions.

When considering low libido, it is important that a full psychological and sexual history is obtained before administering treatment (covered in Chapter 7).

Self-respect

A person who feels unworthy, unattractive or depressed, or who has lost interest in sex, will be unlikely to respond to sexual advances from their partner. Conversely, any woman who feels good about her appearance, is confident and self-assured, and has a positive outlook is more likely to respond positively to sexual advances and compliments.

Partner

It is extremely important that a woman has a high opinion of her partner. Some partners may be unattractive, dull, aggressive or demanding, while others may appear caring, loving and personable. Clearly, individual preference for a partner is diverse, but it is vital that each partner in the couple carefully assesses their contribution to the relationship rather than what they gain from it. Individuals should always be aware of the effect that they can have on their partner in this regard.

Somatic aspects

The clitoris, vulva, vagina, breasts and nipples have long been known to contain erogenous 'zones' that, when appropriately stimulated, produce a pleasurable sexual feeling. However, of greater importance are those little-understood areas of the brain that, when stimulated, result in an erotic response to a variety of sensory and psychological influences. The effects of estrogen, progesterone and testosterone on these regions may have a profound influence on the sexual behavior of some women.

Symptoms of hormone deficiency

Estrogen maintains the integrity of sexual tissues. Following menopause, the vaginal epithelium becomes thin and alkaline, ceases to produce glycogen, shrinks, and is easily damaged or infected. Pelvic fascia loses its elasticity, and the bladder is unable to hold as much urine as when it was more elastic and distensible. The labia become smaller and may flatten completely. Breast glands and alveoli begin to atrophy and are replaced by fat.

Estrogen deficiency may result in marked dyspareunia, vaginal infections, increasing pelvic discomfort and vaginal prolapse. Women often find sexual intercourse extremely uncomfortable and consider their genital region to be unattractive and distasteful to their partner. This combination of physical and psychological influences can result in a complete loss of libido and avoidance of intercourse, often resulting in increased conflict between partners.

Testosterone affects the skin, labia and clitoris, as well as specific cells in the brain. The ovaries of young menstruating women produce testosterone in large amounts, although 93–97% is converted to estradiol. The remaining 3–7% is secreted into the circulation. Most of this testosterone is bound to sex-hormone-binding globulin (SHBG) and is not available for cell activity, but the remaining free testosterone plays a significant role in a woman's sexual response. Following the menopause, ovarian production of testosterone ceases and the only testosterone available to women is the result of conversion of adrenal androstenedione to testosterone. For the majority of women, this may be insufficient.

Key points – sexuality

- Self-respect: a woman who feels she is fat, ugly, unworthy or rejected is unlikely to respond to sexual overtures from her partner.
- Loss of respect for the partner because of physical, psychological or emotional upset can result in sexual rejection.
- A dry atrophic vagina causing severe dyspareunia will inhibit the prospect of enjoyable intercourse.
- Hormone therapy should improve vaginal elasticity and lubrication, and clitoral and nipple sensitivity.
- Low levels of testosterone in women are often found to be associated with loss of libido.

Key references

Davis S. Androgen treatment in women. *Med J Aust* 1999;170: 545–9.

Frock J, Money J. Sexuality and menopause. *Psychother Psychosom* 1992;57:29–33.

Robertson R. Sexuality and the Menopause. In: Wren BG, Nachtigall LE, eds. *Clinical Management of the Menopause.* Sydney: McGraw–Hill, 1996: chapter 5.

In the perimenopause, women usually produce ovarian hormones in a very erratic manner. Often these women are found to have symptoms while their serum estrogen levels are still around premenopausal levels. Alternatively, they can be asymptomatic but have elevations of blood FSH that are suggestive of the menopausal state. Many of these women will also experience irregular bleeding. Changes in the woman's menstrual cycle are often the first sign of an impending menopause and can occur up to 5 years before menstruation actually ceases. Because menstrual irregularity is so prevalent in this group of individuals, low-dose contraceptive therapy is preferred over HT. When women achieve their last spontaneous menstrual period and are, on the basis of symptoms and physical findings, postmenopausal, HT is the principal treatment modality.

The aim of HT is to restore or maintain activity in responsive tissues so that they function more as they did premenopausally. By doing this, it is argued that one can reduce symptoms and maintain quality of life in postmenopausal women.

Before prescribing any HT, a full medical history and physical examination should be performed. Evaluation should include details of prior menstrual cycles including premenstrual-syndrome-type symptoms, conditions such as hepatitis, cancer, thrombosis and cardiovascular problems, and the length of time since last menstruation. The physical examination should be aimed at evaluating vital signs such as blood pressure, height, and weight, as well as breast and pelvic examinations.

Perhaps most important in the current climate of concern regarding use of HT (see Chapter 11, Risks of hormone therapy) is the willingness of the physician to counsel the patient regarding the risk–benefit ratio of HT based on current studies.

The following sections address the management of specific symptoms.

Vasomotor function

Hormone therapy. All hormone preparations have been found to reduce significantly the frequency and severity of hot flashes compared with placebo. The lowest dose of HT should be the initial starting point, and the woman should be re-evaluated after 3 months. If her symptoms are adequately controlled, then that dose of estrogen or estrogen plus progestogen should be continued. If the symptoms are not adequately controlled, then the doses of estrogen or estrogen plus progestogen can be increased. The addition of a progestational agent to the estrogen has been found to have a synergistic effect, with a greater impact on vasomotor symptoms.

It is particularly important that HT is offered to all women having their ovaries removed, even those who are close to the menopause, because of their high risk of developing distressing flashes. Community studies suggest that many women are not currently being offered this choice.

Clonidine, an antihypertensive agent, has been used to treat flashes. It was shown to be more effective than placebo in one randomized controlled clinical trial, but three other trials have not confirmed this. Overall, the response is unpredictable.

Serotonin agonists, such as venlafaxine, have been shown to reduce menopausal flashes and may be particularly suitable for use by women in whom estrogen is to be avoided.

Osteoporosis

There is good evidence that, whatever bone-preserving therapy is used, the effect occurs mainly during treatment and will have diminished significantly within a few years of stopping treatment. An effective osteoporosis treatment strategy will therefore probably involve therapy near the time of greatest need. In relation to hip fracture, this implies treatment relatively late in life, and at this time many favor the use of bisphosphonates. If bone-preserving treatment is given in the early postmenopausal years, it is unlikely to affect later fracture risk, unless continued for many years. Recent trial evidence from a large prospective randomized clinical trial of HT (the WHI trial – see Table 11.2, page 70) confirms that HT can reduce fractures, but there has been criticism that the necessary long-term, or later-life, use of HT is associated with risks that render it second line to bisphosphonates in those circumstances. This question is a matter of ongoing controversy amongst experts, particularly for women who have had a hysterectomy, since the WHI study has indicated that for these women the HT risk profile is less serious.

Hormone therapy. Epidemiological studies have shown that women who have ever used HT have a lower risk of hip fracture than women who have never had HT. Current evidence from the WHI study found a significant reduction in the incidence of hip fracture and in total fractures, an effect demonstrable even in women who were not osteoporotic, whereas the important trials of other agents have mainly selected women with osteoporosis.

Raloxifene is the first selective estrogen-receptor modulator (SERM) to be licensed and has been shown in trials to reduce bone loss at the spine, wrist and hip. However, while a significant reduction in spinal fractures has been demonstrated, no reduction in hip fractures has been seen.

Bisphosphonates are synthetic minerals that become incorporated into the pyrophosphate of the bone mineral, rendering it more resistant to resorption. There is a consequent reduction in bone turnover. There is good evidence from randomized trials that bisphosphonates are effective in the prevention of hip fracture, but this evidence is derived from the study of osteoporotic women in the later postmenopausal years. For this population, bisphosphonates have come to be regarded as the principal option for treatment of osteoporosis. We do not have the same evidence to support the use of bisphosphonates in premenopausal women or in the early postmenopause. Bisphosphonates have also been shown to be effective in the treatment of glucocorticoid-induced osteoporosis.

Etidronate, alendronate and risedronate are the most widely available bisphosphonates.

Etidronate has been available longest and is licensed in many countries for the prevention and treatment of osteoporosis. The licensed regimen in the UK and the USA (used off-label) is a 90-day cycle, with the patient taking etidronate for 14 days and calcium on the other 76 days. The regimens differ in other countries, with 4 weeks of etidronate and 8 weeks of calcium commonly used in Australia. This pattern of administration minimizes the risk of a demineralizing effect on bone. Etidronate tends to be relatively free of side effects when taken cyclically, and 7-year follow-up data in bone density studies have confirmed its effectiveness.

Alendronate has a wider margin between efficacy and any potential demineralization effect, and it can therefore be taken continuously. Alendronate is associated with esophageal irritation, and patients should be advised about strategies to minimize this risk. Generally, the side-effect profile is minimized by the use of the once-weekly oral preparation. The Fracture Intervention Trial has shown that alendronate significantly reduces the risk of fracture in women with established osteoporosis. Recent evidence suggests that after 5 years of alendronate therapy, bone mass may be maintained for several years even after treatment is discontinued.

Risedronate shows similar therapeutic characteristics to alendronate but may be associated with reduced gastrointestinal side effects. As with alendronate, a large randomized trial has shown a significant reduction in hip fractures in osteoporotic women. A once-weekly preparation is available.

Calcitonin is a peptide produced by the thyroid gland; it reduces bone turnover and arrests postmenopausal bone loss. There is also evidence that calcitonin has an analgesic effect on pain associated with osteoporosis. Nasal spray is the most convenient delivery option for calcitonin. In many countries, calcitonin is available only by injection, which limits its use.

Parathyroid hormone is becoming licensed for use in osteoporosis. It differs from the other licensed treatments in that it is able to stimulate bone formation, whereas the other options are antiresorptive. Trials have demonstrated that increases in bone mass and reductions in fracture rates are achieved. This treatment is given by daily injection; it is likely to be an option for use in patients at particularly high risk of fracture.

Other options include the use of calcium supplements, if dietary intake is inadequate, and vitamin D, if exposure to sunlight is limited. Vitamin D is particularly important for elderly women living in nursing homes, and there is good trial evidence of reduced fracture rates in such women when given calcium and vitamin D supplements. For postmenopausal women in general, the use of calcium supplements alone to prevent osteoporosis will be less effective than the options discussed above. Many studies suggest that the rate of bone loss will be reduced, but that overall bone loss will still occur.

Urogenital atrophy

The local symptoms of urogenital atrophy – burning, itching or dryness in the vulvar area, and failure to lubricate at the time of sexual arousal – can be relieved using oral or vaginal estrogen preparations. Estrogen replacement is unlikely to resolve an incontinence problem if there is an anatomic defect for which surgery is required. With oral estrogen or estrogen plus progestogen, approximately 40% of women continue to have vaginal and vulvar symptoms, necessitating the concomitant administration of a local estrogen preparation. The local estrogen can be administered via a tablet, ring or cream.

The response of the vulva or vagina to hormones can be monitored using the vaginal maturation index (percentage of superficial cells). Women who have low estrogen levels have no superficial cells on a vaginal smear taken from the lateral vaginal wall. A dose-related increase in the presence of superficial cells has been observed in women receiving estrogen therapy.

Alternative approaches. There is some evidence that continued sexual activity maintains vaginal blood flow, which helps to minimize the effect of estrogen loss. Currently, there are several lubricating creams and gels available, as well as yogurt preparations. These are of some benefit, but the available clinical evidence is relatively limited.

In cases of stress incontinence, physiotherapy can help to strengthen the pelvic floor, but many women will require pelvic surgery. If there is any diagnostic uncertainty, the use of urodynamic investigation is important.

Neurological function

Cognitive impairment. Most studies to date have indicated that HT increases recall ability for simple things such as verbal and visual information in recently postmenopausal women. In one study, older women were not found to have any change in cognitive function with HT. However, the women who took part in this study were over the age of 65 at entry, and may have already had undetected cognitive decline. The deterioration in cognitive function (probable Alzheimer's disease) occurs principally in women over the age of 75.

Alzheimer's disease. HT has not been shown to have any significant efficacy for the management of established Alzheimer's disease.

Debate continues on the use of HT at an early age to prevent the occurrence of Alzheimer's disease. Observational studies have indicated that the early use of HT (immediately after menopause) appears to reduce the incidence of Alzheimer's disease by 30%. In the WHI memory study (WHIMS), HT did not show any protective effect against probable Alzheimer's disease in women over 65, and there was evidence of an increased risk of developing the condition after 2 years of HT. It could be argued that the increased amount of dementia in WHIMS was due to an increase in atherosclerotic microvascular thrombosis, but the matter is currently unclear.

Sexuality

The loss of libido that often occurs in postmenopausal women can be due to a variety of causes – depression, stress, and family/personal dynamics can all be factors (see Chapter 6). It is important that an in-depth history is taken to try to determine whether there are causes other than the menopause. Using selective serotonin-reuptake inhibitors (SSRIs) can, for example, result in a significant decline in libido in women.

The use of an estrogen can improve sexual interest in postmenopausal women. There is some conflict of ideas regarding the use of testosterone to improve libido, but several well-conducted studies have demonstrated that women with low levels of free testosterone, indicated by a low free androgen index (FAI) and a low libido, see considerable improvement when given appropriate amounts of testosterone. FAI is determined as:

$$\frac{\text{Testosterone level (nmol/liter)} \times 100}{\text{Sex-hormone-binding globulin level (nmol/liter)}} = \text{free androgen index}$$

It is important to appreciate that testosterone given to women with normal FAI levels has not resulted in an increase in sexual desire. As a trial for women with a low FAI, testosterone, 100 mg, can be injected every 2–3 weeks for 6–9 weeks. If there is no improvement after that period, then further use of testosterone should be abandoned. Testosterone can be given on a regular basis as an oral tablet, an implant under the skin, a cream, a patch or a transbuccal troche. Studies using transdermal testosterone have shown limited improvement in only a few areas of sexuality, the most important one being that of visual imagery, which is associated with arousal. Oral methyltestosterone has not been unequivocally shown to improve libido in postmenopausal women. Testosterone pellets have been used, but there is a paucity of information as to their efficacy in terms of improving libido. The use of excessive androgen therapy – oral, transdermal or implants – carries with it the potential for adverse outcomes and side effects such as changes in the voice, increasing hair growth on the face, acne and oily skin.

43

Key points – symptom management

- Hormone therapy (HT) is indicated to improve the quality of life of postmenopausal women.
- HT is not indicated as primary treatment to reduce osteoporosis, cardiovascular disease or Alzheimer's disease.
- A bonus for women taking HT may be a reduction in other diseases.
- For women with a low free androgen index, testosterone may prove beneficial.

Key references

Anderson GL, Limacher M, Assaf AR et al. Women's Health Initiative Steering Committee. Effects of conjugated equine estrogen in postmenopausal women with hysterectomy. *JAMA* 2004;291; 1701–12.

Osteoporosis

Cauley JA, Robbins J, Chen Z et al. Women's Health Initiative Investigators Effects of estrogen plus progestin on risk of fracture and bone mineral density. *JAMA* 2003; 290:1729–38.

Harris ST. Bisphosphonates for the treatment of postmenopausal osteoporosis: clinical studies of etidronate and alendronate. *Osteoporos Int* 2001;12(suppl 3): S11–S16.

Marcus R, Wong M, Heath H, Stock JL. Antiresorptive treatment of postmenopausal osteoporosis: comparison of study designs and outcomes in large clinical trials with fracture as an endpoint. *Endocr Rev* 2002;23:16–37.

McClung MR, Geusens P, Miller PD et al. Effect of risedronate on the risk of hip fracture in elderly women. Hip Intervention Program Study Group. *N Engl J Med* 2001;344:333–40.

Royal College of Physicians. *Osteoporosis: Clinical Guidelines on Prevention and Treatment*. London: Royal College of Physicians, 1999.

Storm T, Kollerup G, Thamsborg G et al. Five years of clinical experience with intermittent cyclical etidronate for postmenopausal osteoporosis. *J Rheumatol* 1996;23:1560–4.

Tilyard MW, Spears GF, Thomson J et al. Treatment of postmenopausal osteoporosis with calcitriol or calcium. *N Engl J Med* 1992;326: 357–62.

Urogenital symptoms

Fantl JA, Cardozo L, McClish DK. Estrogen therapy in the management of urinary incontinence in postmenopausal women: a meta-analysis. *Obstet Gynecol* 1994; 83:12–18.

Raz R, Stamm WE. A controlled trial of intravaginal estriol in postmenopausal women with recurrent urinary tract infections. *N Engl J Med* 1993;329:753–6.

Smith P, Heimer G, Lindskog M et al. Oestradiol-releasing vaginal ring for treatment of postmenopausal urogenital atrophy. *Maturitas* 1993; 16:145–54.

Neurological function

Espeland MA, Rapp SR, Shumaker SA et al. Women's Health Initiative Memory Study. Conjugated equine estrogens and global cognitive function in postmenopausal women. *JAMA* 2004;291:2959–68.

Shumaker SA, Legault C, Kuller L et al. Women's Health Initiative Memory Study. Conjugated equine estrogens and incidence of probable dementia and mild cognitive impairment in postmenopausal women. *JAMA* 2004;291:2947–58.

Shumaker SA, Legault C, Rapp SR et al. Women's Health Initiative Memory Study. Estrogen plus progestin and the incidence of dementia and mild cognitive impairment in postmenopausal women: the Women's Health Initiative Memory Study: a randomized controlled trial. *JAMA* 2003;289:2651–2662.

Sexuality

Davis SR. Androgen treatment in women. *Med J Aust* 1999;170: 545–9.

Sherwin BN, Gelfand MM, Brender W. Androgen enhances sexual motivation in females: a prospective crossover study of sex steroid administration in surgical menopause. *Psychosom Med* 1997;47:339–51.

HT consists of estrogen or, for women with an intact uterus, estrogen plus progestogen (EPT). There are a number of sequential (estrogen followed by progestogen) and continuous combined (estrogen plus progestogen) hormonal preparations available. These provide excellent symptom relief and can be used in almost all postmenopausal women. HT is available as oral tablets, transdermal delivery systems, subdermal implants, nasal sprays, transbuccal troches and vaginal tablets, creams and rings. Side effects associated with one route of administration or dose could require a change in the treatment regimen.

Guidance on the use of HT has recently been published by the International Menopause Society and the North America Menopause Society.

Estrogen plus progestogen regimens

Sequential EPT comprises estrogen for 21 to 31 days each month, with a progestogen added for 12 to 14 days during the last part of the estrogen cycle. This regimen usually results in regular withdrawal bleeding lasting 3 to 4 days.

Combined intermittent EPT is an estrogen and progestogen taken concomitantly for 21 to 25 days with a break of 5 to 7 days. A slight endometrial bleed each month should be anticipated.

Long-interval therapy is the use of an estrogen for 12 weeks with a progestogen added during the last 2 weeks. This can result in heavier endometrial bleeding, but the bleeding occurs only four times a year.

Continuous combined EPT is an estrogen and progestogen taken together every day, with no interval without medication. This is found to reduce bleeding and other menstrually related side effects.

This type of therapy has been used principally for women who are definitely postmenopausal. Women who are more than 3 years postmenopausal appear to have less irregular bleeding during the initiation of continuous combined EPT compared with more recently postmenopausal women. Since there is no anticipated endometrial bleeding with this regimen, a potential advantage is increased patient compliance. Postmenopausal women have been reported to discontinue EPT because of the regular withdrawal bleeding experienced with intermittent or sequential preparations.

The individual patient should be counseled that there could be an increased risk of breakthrough bleeding during the initial 3 to 6 months of continuous combined EPT. The initial spotting that often occurs in women during continuous combined EPT should not be considered clinically important. Only women with heavy bleeding that lasts for several days should have further investigations. All prospective clinical trials of continuous combined EPT have found a low incidence of endometrial hyperplasia (< 1%) and no increase in endometrial cancer, approximately 1 per 7000 women per year. The problem is to distinguish this iatrogenic or HT-related bleeding from neoplasia, which is difficult clinically.

The patient should be counseled that one in every eight women does not achieve amenorrhea or spotting. These patients may require the use of a sequential regimen for anything from 6 to 12 months, or they may need a brief period of time without HT. Continuous combined EPT should be re-initiated after this, with the expectation of limited or no bleeding or spotting.

If the progestogen is started at the same time as the estrogen, the dose of progestogen required to inhibit mitosis and prevent endometrial growth is significantly lower than that required following an estrogen-induced proliferation. The progestogen dose that will inhibit endometrial proliferation is also lower than that needed to induce a secretory change, according to published studies.

Estrogens

Oral estrogens are available as precursor molecules designed to avoid rapid metabolism before reaching the target organ, or they can be identical to the normal female estradiol produced by the functioning ovary. Examples of synthesized estrogen within a stabilized molecule include ethinyl estradiol, estradiol valerate, esterified estrogens and piperazine estrone sulfate. Natural estrogen, such as 17β estradiol, estrone and estriol, is metabolized extensively in the intestinal tract and by the liver. This means that large doses are needed to achieve adequate blood levels when they are given orally. 17β estradiol, when delivered transdermally or intravaginally, is less rapidly metabolized because it bypasses the intestinal tract and the first-pass effect on the liver. Conjugated equine estrogen (CEE) is a mixture of over 100 compounds, but the principal steroid is estrone sulfate.

Commercial preparations. Oral estrogens include CEE (0.3, 0.45, 0.625 or 1.25 mg daily); estradiol valerate (1 or 2 mg daily); piperazine estrone sulfate (0.625, 1.25 or 2.5 mg daily), 17β estradiol (0.5, 1.0 or 2.0 mg daily); and esterified estrogens (0.625 and 1.25 mg daily). 17β estradiol is also available for transdermal administration in patches, creams or gels. 17β estradiol as a pure crystalline pellet is available as a subcutaneous implant. Creams, tablets and rings containing 17β estradiol and CEE have been widely used for their local effect on the vaginal epithelium and the pelvic fascia.

Women who have an intact uterus require a dose of estrogen that will control symptoms, and a progestogen should be used to prevent adverse effects on the endometrium. Lower doses of estrogen and progestogen are now available that meet these criteria.

Oral estrogens stimulate hepatic cholesterol receptors and elevate hepatic lipases, resulting in a reduction in the level of circulating LDL cholesterol. They are easily administered and cost-effective. Oral estrogens can increase hepatic protein synthesis and thus increase the levels of SHBG, thyroid-binding globulin and cortisol-binding globulin. They can also increase the levels of some of the coagulation factors produced by the liver. Oral estrogens are frequently associated with nausea, though rarely with vomiting.

There is an increase in the serum estrogen level for 4 to 6 hours following ingestion of the estrogen, with a fall over the subsequent 12 to 18 hours (Figure 8.1). This rapid absorption followed by a decline may be the reason for such side effects as gastrointestinal upsets following the oral administration. The possible increase in the frequency of migraine headaches may be related to the decline in serum estrogen levels.

Transdermal delivery systems. Transdermal estrogen, principally 17β estradiol, obviously avoids the first-pass liver metabolism and is not degraded by the gastrointestinal tract. This product results in relatively constant blood levels, and has minimal gastrointestinal side effects. There is a reduced stimulation of the cholesterol receptors and lipases in the liver that result in minimal changes in HDL and LDL cholesterol compared with oral formulations. A recent study demonstrated that oral estrogen is associated with a risk of thromboembolism 3.5 times greater than in untreated women, whereas for transdermal estrogen the risk is 0.9. For that reason, women at risk of thrombosis should be encouraged to use a transdermal regimen rather than an oral preparation. There is always a possibility of local skin reactions, due principally to the adhesive, as well as the potential problem of skin adherence. These skin-related problems are minimized with use of a percutaneous gel.

The first-generation transdermal systems contained 17β estradiol in a reservoir of ethanol. 17β estradiol passed through a semipermeable membrane from the reservoir to reach the skin.

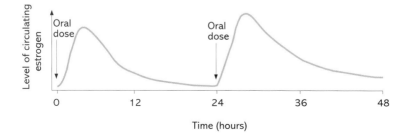

Figure 8.1 The pharmacokinetic profile of oral estrogen.

Newer transdermal systems employ a matrix formulation with the 17β estradiol dissolved in the adhesive material. Some transdermal systems require twice-weekly application, while others need to be changed only once a week owing to their pharmacokinetic profile.

Natural 17β estradiol is also administered in the form of cream or gel. Systemic levels of hormones can be delivered using a percutaneous gel. The application of the alcohol-based gel to the skin allows excellent absorption, and the serum levels of estrogen achieved are related to the surface area of the skin covered with the gel. The gel is a reasonable alternative to the transdermal patches and does not have the same incidence of skin reactions. Gels and creams do require a daily application to maintain the skin reservoir of hormone, however.

Vaginal estrogens. The vaginal epithelium provides an effective absorbing surface. The vagina has a large surface area, so it is possible to achieve significant systemic blood levels using intravaginal estrogen. Several of the vaginal preparations that have been used for many years, such as creams containing CEE or 17β estradiol, are systemically absorbed at standard vaginal doses, so the dose of such preparations can be dramatically reduced while symptom relief is maintained. They should be used only for local effects rather than in an attempt to achieve a significant systemic absorption and management of menopausal symptoms. These statements may not be applicable to estriol cream because of its weak estrogenic activity.

There is a potential for endometrial hyperplasia when vaginal estrogens are used unopposed in women with a uterus, although the clinical data on this are limited. The theoretical possibility exists that vaginally administered estrogens may be preferentially concentrated in the endometrium because of local delivery via vaginal and uterine blood vessels. Therefore, it is appropriate to use a 2-week course of a synthetic progestogen at regular intervals to counteract any endometrial estrogenic effects.

Vaginal rings and tablets are used to administer very-low-dose estradiol for local treatment of the atrophic vaginal epithelium.

Products such as the low-dose vaginal tablet (Vagifem) and the low-dose vaginal ring (Estring) relieve vaginal symptoms without apparent endometrial stimulation or bleeding, so with these therapies progestogens are not administered to protect the endometrium. Vaginal rings delivering larger amounts of 17β estradiol acetate are available for the management of menopausal symptoms. The estradiol acetate vaginal rings that control menopausal symptoms should be used with a progestogen in women with an intact uterus. The systemic levels of 17β estradiol achieved with 17β estradiol acetate rings are high enough to manage the menopausal symptoms, and could result in endometrial stimulation.

Estradiol implants. Natural 17β estradiol has been produced as a crystalline pellet that can be inserted subdermally into the front of the lower abdomen or into the buttock. The implants are usually available in sizes of 20 or 25 mg (depending on the country), 50 mg and 100 mg. These pellets allow 17β estradiol to be slowly released into the circulation. The serum concentration depends not only on the blood supply around the pellet, but on the site of the implant and the surface area of the pellet. The fibrous capsule formed by the body to encase the pellet appears to function as a rate-limiting membrane.

The absorption of estradiol from the implant can be highly variable in terms of the amount and duration of delivery. In some instances, the implants may continue to provide adequate 17β estradiol serum levels for up to 5 years after insertion. In general, though, the circulating serum level of estradiol falls below the maintenance level after 3 to 4 months in the case of 25 mg pellets and at 18 months with 100 mg pellets. In practice, one 50 mg or two 20 mg estradiol implants (40 mg in total) are inserted at 6-month intervals, or 100 mg implants about once a year.

Some women who are using estrogen pellets may continue to complain of hot flashes, sweats and psychological symptoms in spite of having more than adequate serum estradiol levels on testing. This is thought to be due to a tachyphylaxis or a resistance of the hypothalamic thermal regulatory center to continuous levels of estrogen. Some physicians have used progestogens to counteract the effect of estrogen, while others have tried the administration of SSRIs such as fluoxetine or paroxetine. In general, regardless of the therapy used, the estradiol levels must be allowed to return to the normal postmenopausal level before re-initiating therapy. This may result in an unhappy patient, but she can be managed with some of the newer SSRIs or selective serotonin–norepinephrine-reuptake inhibitors for her hot flashes while awaiting a significant reduction in the serum estrogen level. There is evidence that SSRIs can cause excessive perspiration in women. The patient's report of excessive perspiration should be differentiated from a hot flash.

Progestogens

Progesterone or synthetic progestogens have been added to the therapeutic regimens of oral, transdermal and vaginal estrogens in order to prevent endometrial proliferation, endometrial hyperplasia and endometrial cancer in women who have an intact uterus. Progestogens used to be administered for 7 to 10 days, overlapping with estrogen given for 21 days. It has been reported that this amount of progestogen is insufficient to prevent endometrial hyperplasia and endometrial carcinoma. Because of this, the treatment regimen for any progestogen has been extended to 12 to 14 days of each calendar month. This is believed to be optimal to inhibit mitosis, induce a secretory endometrial change, reduce the thickness of the endometrium, and produce a regular shedding or menstruation from the endometrium. More recent evidence has suggested that using a 12-day cycle of progestogen therapy for more than 5 years may result in an increased incidence of endometrial cancer. Current data indicate that continuous combined EPT, when used over 4 to 5 years, can result in a significant reduction in the incidence of endometrial cancer relative to that in women who have never used HT.

Natural progesterone taken orally is rapidly metabolized. Because of this, the serum level of progesterone is usually variable or low after an oral dose.

'Natural' (bio-identical) progesterone is manufactured using multiple enzymatic activities on a substrate (diosgenin) found in wild yams and Chinese yews. It is available as both oral and transdermal preparations. When manufactured under strict procedures, bio-identical progesterone taken orally has been shown to produce reasonable blood levels that are able to convert the endometrium to a secretory or atrophic pattern and to prevent the development of hyperplasia and adenocarcinoma. The manufacture of transdermal progesterone creams is currently unregulated, and the serum progesterone levels that are achieved are less than adequate to protect the endometrium.

Synthetic progestogens have been manufactured in order to overcome the problem of variable serum levels. They maintain a positive response on the endometrium by inhibiting estrogen receptors and the proliferative activity of estrogen. As part of their biological activity, progestogens cause a morphologic change in the endometrium to a secretory histological pattern. They include a variety of steroid types, and can be derived from progesterone itself, from 17α-hydroxyprogesterone molecules, or from a 19-nortestosterone substrate. The 19-nortestosterone progestational agents are more potent in terms of their endometrial activity per mg administered, but are more likely to induce androgenic side effects such as acne or oily skin. Progestogens derived from C-21 steroids have been reported to produce more changes in somatic symptoms. The appropriate progestogen for a patient requires individualization based on the clinical response (side effects).

Key points – types of hormone therapy

- Estrogen may be administered by the oral, transdermal, subdermal, nasal, transbuccal or vaginal route.
- Bio-identical natural progesterone is rapidly metabolized by enzymes in the gut and liver.
- Synthetic progestogens are stable and effective orally, transdermally and as an intrauterine device.
- Regimens of therapy should be tailored to the needs of individual women.

Key references

British Menopause Society. *BMS Council Consensus Statement on Hormone Replacement Therapy.* June 2004. www.the-bms.org/consensus.htm

International Menopause Society. Guidelines for hormone treatment of women in the menopausal transition and beyond Position Statement by the Executive Committee of the International Menopause Society [revised 15 October 2004]. *Climacteric* 2004;7:333–7. www.imsociety.org/PDF/news_IMS_statement_15.10.04.pdf?PHPSESSID=5c0fdb961379784326119d3c3fcb2c04

North American Menopause Society. Recommendations for estrogen and progestogen use in peri- and postmenopausal women: October 2004 position statement of The North American Menopause Society. *Menopause* 2004;11:589–600. www.menopause.org/edumaterials/2004HTreport.pdf

Rees M, Purdie DW, eds. *Management of the Menopause,* 3rd edn. Marlow: BMS Publications, 2002.

Scarabin PY, Oger E, Plu-Bureau G; EStrogen and THromboEmbolism Risk Study Group. Differential association of oral and transdermal oestrogen-replacement therapy with venous thromboembolism risk. *Lancet* 2003;362:428–32.

Common side effects that have been associated with HT are shown in Table 9.1. The significant adverse events that have been associated with HT are discussed in Chapter 11.

Bloating

Progestogens have been found to have an inhibitory effect on the motility of smooth muscle. Women who use progestational agents have been found to have slow peristalsis of the gastrointestinal tract, occasional urinary retention, and a potential increase in the occurrence of gallstones. Food stays in the gastrointestinal tract for longer, leading to an increase in bloating, constipation and intestinal gas. In some instances, it has been argued that the progestogens increase weight because of water retention or edema. Stasis of bile in the gallbladder may result in an increase in gallstone formation, and cholecystitis has been reported in women using estrogens.

To some extent, the intestinal bloating can be controlled by reducing the dose of the progestogen, changing to a different progestogen, or even by using a transdermal formulation of the progestogen. There are limited data on transdermal compared with oral progestogens. It is reasonable to assume that the progestogen dose that elicits a secretory change in the endometrium will also

TABLE 9.1

Common side effects associated with hormone therapy

- Bloating
- Edema
- Mastalgia
- Skin changes, acne
- Endometrial spotting/bleeding
- Headaches, migraine

have a comparable effect in other target tissues in the body. However, this is more of a hypothesis than a reflection of known clinical information.

Edema

Edema or puffiness of the lower extremities associated with HT is generally due to poor circulation in the leg. It can be caused by venous stasis resulting from varicose veins, or venous obstruction, with increasing hydrostatic back pressure related to sitting or standing in one position for a long period of time, or a local reactive process. Lymphatic obstruction from a variety of causes can also result in edema.

Edema in the lower extremities that disappears during the night is probably not hormonally related. This is more likely to be due to a stasis or gravitational effect or secondary to prolonged standing. Estrogen may lead to a reduction in the extracellular escape of fluid by improving the arterial endothelium and it also probably has other effects on the capillaries. Investigations of the levels of electrolytes during HT have consistently failed to demonstrate any imbalance. Women who experience peripheral edema should be encouraged to exercise or to use an isometric tightening of the muscles when standing on their feet and to elevate their feet when sitting or resting. Persistent edema that is of clinical significance can be treated with diuretics.

Mastalgia

It is important to understand that estrogen not only increases the rate of mitosis of breast cells, but it is also responsible for the induction of both estrogen and progesterone receptors. Progesterone, on the other hand, has a biphasic action on breast cells. Initially it increases mitosis, but later the continual application of progesterone leads to reduction in receptors, inhibition of cell division and maturation of alveolar cells. Because of this maturation, these cells become engorged with the proteins and fluid which is normally involved in secreting milk. Thus the initial effect of progestogen is to induce full, tight breasts. Accordingly, postmenopausal women given an estrogen and/or an estrogen plus progestogen often complain of intense mastalgia (breast pain), which may result in discontinuation of HT. Continuous combined HT has been associated with mastalgia principally in the first 3 months of treatment. With time, the incidence of breast discomfort is reduced. In some instances, switching from a continuous combined therapy to a cyclic therapy may be beneficial. Reducing the dose of the estrogen and/or progestogen has been found to lower the incidence of mastalgia significantly. Mastalgia is also present in women using transdermal HT.

The use of the progestogen first before estrogen has been found to result in an increase in breast secretory activity, but this is then followed by an inhibition of mitosis and a remission of pain. It is possible, with counseling and reassurance over a period of 1 to 2 months, that women will be willing to accept the mild to moderate mastalgia. In some women, mastalgia is persistent and is so uncomfortable that discontinuation of HT may be advised. Postmenopausal women who present with mastalgia should be reassured that this symptom is not associated with cancer.

Progestogens have been found to increase breast-cell differentiation and mitotic activity in the premenopausal woman. Recent clinical reports suggest that progestogen may be involved in increasing the incidence of breast neoplasia (see Chapter 11).

Skin changes

Acne and oily skin are usually due to androgenic progestogens such as the 19-nor compounds, as exemplified by norethisterone and levonorgestrol. Both progestogens may increase androgenic receptor responses in hair follicles and sebaceous glands. If these side effects are significant, the progestogen should be replaced with either cyproterone acetate or dydrogesterone. Skin changes that are the result of the progestogen are not permanent and will often subside with appropriate intervention.

Obstruction of the hair follicle with detritus and secondary infection with bacteria is commonly associated with androgenic hormones – norethisterone, levonorgestrol and testosterone.

Cyproterone acetate has been a treatment for women who develop acneform pustules. When administered in combination with an estrogen, cyproterone acetate usually results in remission of acne.

Headaches

Non-migraine-type headaches have been associated with progestogens. A small number of women taking a progestogen complain of a dull intermittent headache. Reducing the dose or changing the progestogen may reduce the incidence of headaches. Natural micronized progesterone and the progestogen dydrogesterone appear to produce fewer headaches than nortestosterone derivatives.

Migraine headaches. Over 80% of women with migraines do not have a hormonal basis for their symptoms. In those women who experience migraines while on HT, onset of the headache is usually triggered by a fall in the level of estrogen or progestogen or both. In younger women, this is associated with the end of the ovarian hormonal cycle, and the migraine is called menstrual migraine. Postmenopausal women receiving sequential EPT find that migraines frequently occur during the time when they are not taking either hormone. Postmenopausal women who suffer from migraine are best treated with continuous estrogen alone or continuous estrogen plus progestogen. In some instances, the transdermal administration of a continuous estrogen or estrogen plus progestogen may be even more effective, since it will result in more stable blood levels of hormones than occur with oral administration.

Key points – side effects of hormone therapy

• Progestogens induce most of the adverse events associated with hormone therapy.
• Inhibition of smooth muscle activity and mastalgia are the commonest side effects of progestogen therapy.
• Adverse effects may be managed by reducing the dosage, varying the delivery system or changing the delivery schedule.
• Bio-identical progesterone is rapidly metabolized by enzymes and is therefore unreliable as a therapy option.

Key reference

Wren BG. Transdermal progesterone or synthetic progestogens. *J Brit Menop Soc* 2001;7:115–19.

Bleeding with combination hormone therapy

The cyclic administration of an estrogen plus progestogen (sequential) on a monthly basis or on a 3- or 6-monthly or yearly basis will usually result in withdrawal bleeding episodes. Breakthrough bleeding or irregular bleeding and spotting can occur early in women who have started continuous combined HT. The actual reason for this bleeding in the presence of an atrophic endometrium is unknown. One hypothesis is that the capillaries in the endometrium become more fragile.

Investigation. Ultrasound evaluation of women using continuous combined HT usually confirms that the endometrium stripe is thin. For most individuals, it is rarely necessary to perform a diagnostic curettage. If bleeding persists and is heavy, then further evaluation with a curettage or, in some instances, hysteroscopy is indicated.

Management. For persistent problematic bleeding during continuous combined EPT, stopping and changing to a cyclic regimen should be the first step. Lowering the dose of estrogen and progestogen is a second step and usually results in a decreased incidence of bleeding. Increasing the progestogen dose can be an option, but it is not recommended as immediate treatment.

Bleeding with unopposed estrogen

Unopposed estrogen can cause proliferative changes in the endometrium, including endometrial hyperplasia. Long-term use of unopposed estrogen increases the incidence of endometrial cancer.

Investigation. Any type of endometrial bleeding in a woman receiving unopposed estrogen should be investigated by endometrial curettage. The incidence of endometrial hyperplasia varies based on the type of estrogen and the dosage, but it is 15–20% at the end of 1 year in women taking unopposed estrogen.

Management. If there is no evidence of atypical hyperplasia or carcinoma after evaluation, then therapy consists usually of a 2-week course of an appropriate progestogen. This should be followed with cyclic or continuous progestogen therapy rather than with unopposed estrogen therapy.

Menorrhagia

In a few instances very heavy bleeding, either regular or irregular, can occur during unopposed estrogen therapy or, in some cases, associated with EPT. There is an increased incidence of irregular bleeding in women who have underlying problems such as uterine fibroids. Adenomyosis, endometrial polyps or neoplasia should be considered if the bleeding is profuse and persistent.

Investigation. Diagnostic curettage is often the appropriate choice associated with an ultrasound scan. Ultrasound evaluation of the endometrium can show increased endometrial thickness while women are receiving estrogen plus progestogen. The endometrium frequently has a benign (atrophic) histological appearance. Ultrasound evaluation of the endometrium in women using EPT is not sensitive enough to use as a screening modality. Depending on the result of the clinical evaluation, surgical intervention and/or change in the hormonal therapy may be necessary.

> **Key points – endometrial bleeding with hormone therapy**
>
> • Breakthrough bleeding is relatively common in the early phase of continuous combined hormone therapy.
> • Bleeding should initially be treated by ceasing therapy for a short interval, changing to a sequential therapy or reducing the dosage.
> • Persistent, recurrent bleeding requires investigation.

Key references

Beresford SAA, Weiss NS, Voigt LF et al. Risk of endometrial cancer in relation to use of estrogen combined with cyclic progestogen therapy in postmenopausal women. *Lancet* 1997;349:458–61.

Grady D, Gebretsadik T, Kerlikowske K et al. Hormone replacement therapy and endometrial cancer risk: a meta-analysis. *Obstet Gynecol* 1995;85:304–13.

Woodruff JD, Pickar JH. Incidence of endometrial hyperplasia in postmenopausal women taking conjugated estrogens (Premarin) with medroxyprogesterone acetate or conjugated estrogens alone. The Menopause Study Group. *Am J Obstet Gynecol* 1994;170:1213–23.

There is an extensive debate in the medical community over the incidence of cardiovascular and neoplastic disease and the possible association with HT. These medical issues, which have been picked up by the media, have had a significant impact on acceptability for the patient and on women's continuation of estrogen or EPT. Several major observational studies published over the past few years have contributed to the debate and have caused considerable concern to both doctors and their patients. However, these studies must be carefully evaluated before the findings are accepted as being applicable to all postmenopausal women or all therapy regimens.

In contrast to these observational studies, the WHI trial has the additional validity of being a well-conducted randomized controlled trial, but it is important to emphasize that it was not designed to focus on the effects of HRT in the group of women who have commonly used HRT, namely those in the menopausal transition and in the first postmenopausal decade (say up to 60 years), often for only a few years. Instead, the study was intended to address the effects of HT taken by older postmenopausal women who might use it for an extended number of years for potential long-term health benefit (particularly cardiovascular benefit), an idea becoming popular in the USA at the time the WHI study was designed. This important difference tends to be ignored in the media attention paid to the results of the WHI study, and as a result women in the first postmenopausal decade, who have read headlines about risk, feel concerned about using HT for relief of troublesome symptoms.

Effects of estrogen and estrogen deficiency

Atherosclerosis. Until they reach menopause, women have a markedly reduced risk of atherosclerosis compared with age-matched men. Following menopause, levels of LDL cholesterol increase. LDL cholesterol has a tendency to be deposited in the arterial intima, leading to atherosclerosis, so postmenopausal women develop atherosclerosis at a rate that parallels the rate for men. Estrogen reduces this effect.

Estrogen appears to have several effects that contribute to the prevention of atherosclerosis.

- Estrogen acts as a potent antioxidant to prevent oxidation of LDL cholesterol. Oxidized LDL is toxic to arterial endothelial cells. The toxic damage causes platelets to release a number of mitogenic factors, which make cells within the vessel wall proliferate, and also induce procoagulant activity.
- Estrogen also has a role in maintaining the integrity of the endothelium.
- In addition, estrogen has a major beneficial effect on HDL cholesterol levels.

The consequences of the hardened arterial walls of atherosclerosis include:

- increased blood pressure
- reduced peripheral blood flow
- increased arterial thrombosis
- increased cardiovascular-related mortality.

Thrombosis. The estrogen deficiency following menopause results in increased risk of thrombosis. The three main causes of thrombosis are:

- damage to the vascular endothelium, which is responsible for maintaining normal hemostasis
- stasis of circulating blood
- changes to the coagulation mechanisms, including an imbalance between the factors that favor coagulation and those that induce fibrinolysis.

Genetic defects in the hemostatic system can increase the risk of thrombosis, and it is important to distinguish these effects from that of estrogen deficiency following the menopause. Some 40–50% of women who develop a thromboembolus are subsequently found to have a congenital coagulation defect. Some women (3%) inherit an abnormal Factor V molecule (Factor V Leiden) – this is a coagulating factor that is resistant to activated protein C, an anticoagulant that inactivates Factor V. For women with a family history of Factor V abnormality, the risk of thrombosis may be up to 30-fold higher when using an oral contraceptive.

Other risk factors for thrombosis. Postmenopausal women who have hypertension or varicose veins, smoke, are overweight or lead a sedentary lifestyle are at increased risk of thrombosis.

Vasodilation. Estrogen has been shown to induce vasodilation in both coronary and peripheral arteries. Clinically, this results in:
• increased blood flow
• lower blood pressure
• reduced incidence of angina and claudication
• reduced morbidity and mortality from cardiovascular accidents.
These benefits decline following the menopause.

Estrogen also acts directly on endothelial cells, inducing production of nitric oxide, also known as endothelial-derived relaxing factor (EDRF). EDRF has a known vasodilatory effect, resulting in improved blood flow. This action is diminished following the menopause.

Ventricular output. Progressive enlargement of the heart has been found in postmenopausal women. This is associated with an increase in ventricular wall thickness and a reduction in stroke volume, which increase the risk of ischemic heart disease, myocardial infarction, cardiac failure and ventricular rupture.

The effects of estrogen on the arterial system, cardiac output and blood lipids are summarized in Table 11.1.

In the breast. The breast is composed of a number of diverse hormone-sensitive cell types (Figure 11.1). As pointed out earlier, estrogen increases the rate of mitotic proliferation in both the alveolar and ductal cells, while progestogens are associated with the development and maturation of alveolar cells. Progestogens also initiate change in the alveolar cells that normally precede secretory

TABLE 11.1

The effects of estrogen deficiency and replacement on the cardiovascular system

	Following menopause	Following estrogen replacement
Lipids		
Total cholesterol	Elevated	Reduced
LDL cholesterol	Elevated	Reduced
Lipoprotein (a)	Elevated	Reduced
HDL cholesterol	Reduced	Elevated
Blood pressure	Elevated	Reduced
Peripheral resistance	Increased	Reduced
Left ventricular function		
Muscle mass	Increased	Reduced
Stroke volume	Reduced	Increased
Left ventricular size	Increased	Reduced
Endothelium response		
Endothelium dependent	Endothelin-1 increased	Endothelin-1 reduced
Endothelium independent	Calcium influx increased	Calcium influx reduced
Hemostasis		
Fibrinogen	Reduced	Elevated
Antithrombin III	Unchanged	Unchanged
Proteins C and S	Unchanged	May be elevated
Plasminogen-activating inhibitor-1	Elevated	Reduced
Factor VII	Elevated	Uncertain

HDL, high-density lipoprotein; LDL, low-density lipoprotein.

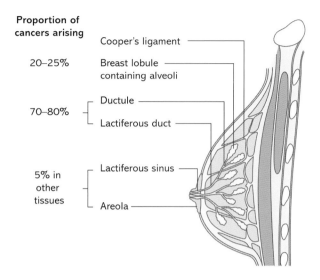

Proportion of cancers arising

Cooper's ligament

20–25%   Breast lobule containing alveoli

70–80%   Ductule

Lactiferous duct

5% in other tissues   Lactiferous sinus

Areola

Figure 11.1 Cross-section of the breast showing the sites at which cancer can occur.

function as well as inducing an inhibitory effect of mitosis on the breast cells.

It is now believed that most of the estrogen that influences breast-cancer-cell activity is derived locally by enzymatic conversion of precursors into estradiol. Breast-cancer cells appear to stimulate surrounding fat cells to increase production of enzymes such as aromatase and sulfatase, which convert androgens or estrone sulfate to estradiol. The level of estrogen in cells surrounding a cancer is 20–30 times higher than in the circulating blood. For this reason, blocking agents such as tamoxifen, raloxifene or enzyme inhibitors such as anastrozole may play a major role in controlling the growth rate of breast-cancer cells. Tibolone inhibits sulfatase activity and therefore may be of value, in conjunction with aromatase inhibitors, in reducing the local production and effect of estrogen.

The effect of hormone therapy

The WHI study is the only major randomized controlled trial of the use of HT in an apparently healthy population of postmenopausal

67

women and, as such, deserves primacy in our assessment of the evidence in this field. The study is summarized in Table 11.2 (pages 70–74). Although, as pointed out above, it was not designed to look especially at the effects of HT in the younger postmenopausal population who are the predominant users of HT, it does nevertheless provide some perspective on that group.

The total WHI study population spanned the three postmenopausal decades from 50 to 79 years and, since the associated risks increase with age irrespective of HT use, it is important to consider what WHI revealed about risk in the specific decade of life that relates to the individual patient. Since the original publication of WHI, detailed papers containing those decade-specific data have appeared. In considering these data, professionals and their patients must understand that, although the data come from the largest randomized controlled trial for the effects of HT for those age groups, the trial size was not sufficient for absolute conclusions to be drawn; if no difference between groups was observed, this could simply mean that the numbers studied, though large, were not large enough to show up any difference.

As described in Table 11.3, the estrogen–progestogen component of WHI provided evidence that combined EPT is associated with a reduced risk of osteoporotic fractures and bowel cancer but a non-significant increased risk of breast cancer, heart attacks and stroke. When published, these figures induced fear among women and warnings of dire consequences from various health professionals, often without any regard to whether the differences observed were statistically significant or not. Two years later the results of the WHI study on use of estrogen alone were published (Table 11.3), and this time the use of CEE was found to be associated with a non-significant reduction in the risk of breast cancer, no significant increase in the risk of cardiovascular disease or thromboembolism and a 39% reduction in osteoporotic fracture but an increased risk of stroke (12/10 000 per year).

The major problem for those who wish to use the WHI data to describe the experience of women in the first postmenopausal decade is that the WHI study dealt with a group of women who were generally older than the group who present with menopausal symptoms. Additionally, those interested in the experience of healthy young postmenopausal women using HT for symptom relief criticize the WHI population as being not ideally 'healthy'. The women in the WHI trial are described as:

- generally free of menopausal symptoms
- having an average age > 63 years, ranging up to 79 years
- overweight, with 34% being obese and only 30% being in the healthy range
- being a current or past smoker (50%)
- having diabetes (4.4%)
- having evidence of prior cardiovascular disease, with 37% requiring therapy for hypertension and 12.5% having pathologically elevated cholesterol levels.

Such a group overall differs from typical symptomatic HT users, but the differences were not explained in the media, and therefore the WHI data caused a degree of panic and avoidance of HT amongst the young postmenopausal group who would have used HT for symptom relief.

The WHI trial is a landmark study because of its scale and duration, and its findings therefore carry particular weight, but debate remains over the extent to which the data can be extrapolated to apply to all forms of HT. WHI employed oral CEE in a continuous combined regimen with medroxyprogestogen acetate. Can all of the outcomes be extrapolated as class effects to all HT? It appears likely that for the skeletal effect this is the case, but there is good evidence from metabolic, mechanistic and animal studies to suggest that different estrogens, different progestogens and different routes of administration produce differences in the cardiovascular effects that result. The relevance of the cardiovascular outcomes of WHI to a woman using a different HT product, and perhaps taking it by a different route, such as transdermally, remains an open question.

TABLE 11.2

Key studies of the effects of hormone therapy (HT)

The Women's Health Initiative (WHI) Study

This landmark randomized controlled trial is by far the largest undertaken. It is effectively two studies, which generally applied the same methodology, one comparing estrogen–progestogen therapy (EPT) with placebo in postmenopausal women and one comparing estrogen with placebo in hysterectomized postmenopausal women. Both studies were terminated early by the data-monitoring committee, the EPT study in 2002, at a mean of 5.2 years, because of criteria based on a global health index and breast cancer outcomes, and the estrogen study in 2004, at a mean of 6.8 years, because of a small increase in stroke risk in a context where the final year of the study was judged unlikely to change the outcomes already established.

Both studies span 30 years after the menopause, a period in which the absolute risk of disease events increases. The 10-year specific absolute risks from the WHI study indicate absolute risk differences due to HT use for each decade, but these estimates should be interpreted with caution, since the study was not powered for these subgroup analyses.

The WHI estrogen study

Design. A randomized controlled trial of intended duration 8.5 years with subsequent follow-up. Terminated at mean duration 6.8 years.

Participants. 10 739 'healthy' postmenopausal women aged 50–79 years who had previous hysterectomy. The women were sufficiently free of menopausal symptoms that they could be randomized to placebo for a span of years.

Interventions
- *Active:* daily oral conjugated equine estrogens, 0.625 mg; n = 5310
- *Control:* daily oral placebo; n = 5429

TABLE 11.2

Key studies of the effects of HT (continued)

Outcomes. The primary outcomes were coronary heart disease (CHD) events, but a wide range of clinical events was studied. The use of conjugated equine estrogens was found to be associated with a non-significant reduction in the risk of breast cancer and CHD and a non-significant increase in thromboembolism, a significant reduction in osteoporotic fracture but an increased risk of stroke.

The WHI estrogen–progestogen study

Design. A randomized controlled trial of intended duration 8.5 years with subsequent follow-up. Terminated at mean duration 5.2 years.

Participants. 16 608 'healthy' postmenopausal women aged 50–79 years who had not had hysterectomy. The women were sufficiently free of menopausal symptoms that they could be randomized to placebo for a span of years.

Interventions
- *Active:* daily oral conjugated equine estrogens, 0.625 mg, and continuous medroxyprogesterone acetate, 2.5 mg; n = 8506
- *Control:* daily oral placebo; n = 8102

Outcomes. The primary outcomes were CHD events, but a wide range of clinical events was studied. Combined EPT was found to be associated with a reduced risk of osteoporotic fractures but a non-significant increased risk of breast cancer, heart attacks and stroke.

References

Anderson GL, Limacher M, Assaf AR et al. Women's Health Initiative Steering Committee. Effects of conjugated equine estrogen in postmenopausal women with hysterectomy. *JAMA* 2004;291:1701–12.

Rassouw JE, Anderson GL, Prentice RL et al. Writing Group for the Women's Health Initiative Investigators. Risks and benefits of estrogen plus progestin in healthy postmenopausal women. *JAMA* 2002;288:321–33.

CONTINUED

TABLE 11.2

Key studies of the effects of HT (continued)

The Heart and Estrogen/Progestin Replacement Study (HERS)

This was the first of the large randomized controlled trials of HT with clinical event end-points. It was designed to test whether further CHD events could be reduced by HT in women with established CHD.

Design. A randomized controlled trial of 4 years' duration with subsequent follow-up.

Participants. 2763 postmenopausal women aged 50–79 years who had previously experienced a coronary heart event.

Interventions

- *Active:* daily oral conjugated equine estrogens, 0.625 mg, plus daily medroxyprogesterone acetate, 2.5mg; n = 1380
- *Control:* daily oral placebo; n = 1383

Outcomes. The primary outcome was CHD death, but other clinical events were studied. In summary, CHD deaths were the same in both groups over 4 years. In the HT group, such deaths were increased in the first year and reduced in the subsequent 3 years, with no overall difference over 4 years. A majority of the women continued, unblinded, on the same therapies up to year 8. Overall a benefit from HT was not found.

References

Grady D, Herrington D, Bittner V et al. Cardiovascular disease outcomes during 6.8 years of hormone therapy. *JAMA* 2002;288:49–57.

Hulley S, Furberg C, Barrett-Connor E et al. Noncardiovascular disease outcomes during 6.8 years of hormone therapy. *JAMA* 2002;288:58–66.

Hulley S, Grady D, Bush T et al. Randomized trial of estrogen plus progestin for secondary prevention of coronary heart disease in postmenopausal women. *JAMA* 1998;280:605–13.

TABLE 11.2

Key studies of the effects of HT (continued)

The Nurses Health Study

This is probably the most famous and important observational study of the long-term effects of HT, and is based on a study of American nurses. It has been a major source of information on the long-term health effects of HT before the HERS and WHI trials.

Design. A cohort study of the health experience of nurses, commenced in 1976 with repeated questionnaire follow-up.

Participants. 122 000 North American nurses aged 30–55 years.

Intervention. Observation of the differences in health experience of users of HT and non-users of HT.

Outcomes. CHD was the primary focus of the study; the results suggested significant benefit from HT use. The study also suggested an increase in breast cancer risk in HT users.

References

Colditz GA, Hankinson SE, Hunter DJ et al. The use of estrogens and progestins and the risk of breast cancer in postmenopausal women. *N Engl J Med* 1995;332:1589–93.

Grodstein F, Stampfer MJ, Manson JE et al. Postmenopausal estrogen and progestin use and the risk of cardiovascular disease. *N Engl J Med* 1996;335:453–61; *N Engl J Med* 1996;335:1406.

Stampfer MJ, Willett WC, Colditz GA et al. A prospective study of postmenopausal estrogen therapy and coronary heart disease. *N Engl J Med* 1985;313:1044–9.

Stampfer MJ, Colditz GA, Willett WC et al. Postmenopausal estrogen therapy and cardiovascular disease. Ten-year follow-up from the nurses' health study. *N Engl J Med* 1991:325;756–62.

CONTINUED

TABLE 11.2

Key studies of the effects of HT (continued)

The Collaborative Group on Hormones and Cancer

This landmark study reanalyzed essentially the whole of the epidemiological literature on HT and breast cancer based on the original data of 51 studies. This reanalysis indicated an association between breast-cancer risk and duration of HT use and resolution of the increased risk after HT use is discontinued, particularly after 5 years.

References

Collaborative Group on Hormonal Factors in Breast Cancer. Breast cancer and hormone replacement therapy: Collaborative reanalysis of data from 51 epidemiological studies of 52 705 women with breast cancer and 108 411 women without breast cancer. *Lancet* 1997;350:1047–59.

TABLE 11.3

Comparison of estrogen alone and estrogen plus progestogen

	Combined (EPT)	Estrogen alone
Breast cancer	Increase of 8/10 000 (NS)	Decrease of 7/10 000 (NS)
Bowel cancer	Decrease of 6/10 000 (NS)	Increase of 1/10 000 (NS)
Uterine cancer	Decrease of 1/10 000 (NS)	– (no uterus)
All fractures	Decrease of 44/10 000	Decrease of 5/10 000
Stroke	Increase of 8/10 000 (NS)	Increase of 12/10 000
Cardiovascular disease	Increase of 7/10 000 (NS)	Decrease of 5/10 000 (NS)
Thrombo-embolism	Increase of 18/10 000	Increase of 7/10 000 (NS)
Symptoms	Decrease of 90%	Decrease of 65%

Risk is stated per year. NS, not significant.
Data from the Women's Health Initiative studies.

Cardiovascular disease. The current debate on the relationship between cardiovascular disease and HT stems from the contrast between the longstanding literature of observational studies, which indicated a reduction of approximately 30% in cardiovascular risk in initially healthy HT users, and the clinical results from two more recent randomized trials, which suggest no benefit (the Heart and Estrogen/Progestin Replacement Study – HERS – and WHI) and in fact have raised the possibility of harm (WHI). The contention is that the incidence of cardiovascular events increases in the first year after initiating HT. The overall outcome in both studies was null: there was no statistically significant change in the incidence of cardiovascular disease in women using HT (Table 11.4).

One hypothesis to explain this discrepancy is that HT initiated at the time of menopause can retard or prevent the development of atherosclerosis, but if there is a gap between the occurrence of menopause and the initiation of HT, then there could be an

TABLE 11.4

Adjusted relative hazard values and 95% confidence intervals for primary cardiovascular disease events in HERS, HERS II and overall

HERS	0.96 (0.78–1.18)
HERS II	0.98 (0.75–1.22)
Overall	0.97 (0.82–1.14)
Year 1	1.51 (1.00–2.27)
Year 2	0.94 (0.63–1.41)
Year 3	0.80 (0.51–1.26)
Year 4	0.56 (0.34–0.92)
Year 5	1.06 (0.69–1.62)
Years 6–8	0.98 (0.72–1.34)

Adjusted for age, ethnicity, smoking, body mass index, diabetes, systolic blood pressure, creatinine clearance, exercise, general health, history of congestive heart failure and myocardial infarction, and baseline use of aspirin, angiotensin-converting enzyme inhibitors and statins and statin use during follow-up.
HERS, Heart and Estrogen/Progestin Replacement Study.
Reproduced with permission from Grady D et al. *JAMA* 2002;288:49–57.

increased occurrence of atherosclerosis. In some women, an atherosclerotic plaque could be significant, and subsequent HT could result in destabilization and thrombosis. Data from human trials using ultrasound imaging of carotid arteries have demonstrated a prevention or retardation of the progression of intima-medial thickness in women at younger ages who use HT. In women with established atherosclerotic plaques with luminal narrowing in the coronary or carotid arteries, the use of HT has not been shown to have any effect on decreasing plaque size compared with placebo. These data have been used to support the contention that once atherosclerotic disease or endothelial cell dysfunction has occurred, HT may be of no benefit.

All of these points could mean that older, apparently healthy women, like those in the WHI trial, are at a different level of risk and have a different, lower, potential benefit from HT than young postmenopausal women. Whatever the basis for the different messages from observational studies and randomized controlled trials, it is clear that HT is not recommended for the secondary prevention of cardiovascular disease. With respect to the primary prevention of coronary heart disease, the possibility that HT initiated at the menopause may maintain coronary health and prevent future disease continues to be debated.

Stroke. Although several studies have seen no increase in the risk of stroke in women using HT, others have reported a slight but statistically significant increase. The current WHI data show an increased incidence of ischemic stroke in HT users compared with those receiving placebo. It should be recalled again, however, that women recruited to the study were several years older than the average woman at menopause, and some had underlying disease processes such as diabetes and hypertension. A subgroup analysis of the WHI data did not show a greater incidence of stroke in women who had underlying disease, were more at risk of stroke and were taking HT than in a matched subgroup taking placebo. Possibly these older, hypertensive women already had damage to vessel endothelium before treatment.

The WHI study showed a marked age effect in the absolute risk of stroke in HT users compared with non-users. In women aged 70–79 years, the increase in stroke was 13 and 14 cases per 10 000 women per year, for EPT and estrogen only, respectively, whereas for the age group who most commonly use HT (50–59 years) the increase in absolute risk of stroke was 4 (EPT) and zero (estrogen only) cases per 10 000 women per year.

A prospective randomized study of women who had had a stroke did not show any increase or decrease in the recurrence of stroke, nor was overall mortality changed in estrogen-only users.

It is important to counsel patients that they may be at increased risk of stroke while using HT, and to present appropriate statistics for the individual's situation.

Hypertension. In general, clinical trials with estrogen or EPT have failed to show any significant effect on either systolic or diastolic blood pressure. If there is any change, it is usually less than 1–2 mmHg in mean systolic or diastolic blood pressure. There have been isolated instances of an idiosyncratic reaction with significant elevation in blood pressure after the use of HT. An important aspect of identifying this is to stop the medication to see if blood pressure normalizes. If blood pressure does not normalize, antihypertensive medication is indicated. Women who are well controlled with antihypertensive medications do not have a contraindication to HT.

Deep-vein thrombosis and pulmonary embolism. Postmenopausal women, as they age, have an increased risk of deep-vein thrombosis. Both observational and prospective randomized clinical trials find an increased incidence of deep-vein thrombosis and pulmonary emboli associated with the use of postmenopausal oral estrogen and progestogen combinations. There are also changes in a variety of coagulation factors in postmenopausal women, some of which are procoagulant and some of which are anticoagulant. There has never been any evidence that these changes in the coagulation factors have any correlation with the occurrence of clinical disease such as venous thromboembolism or pulmonary emboli. It is important to note that coagulation occurs spontaneously only when there has been underlying damage to the vascular endothelium (as with atherosclerosis, trauma, varicose veins and smoking).

Idiopathic deep-vein thrombosis occurs spontaneously in about 1 per 5000 postmenopausal women each year. HT may triple this rate in the first 8 months of use. This risk may persist in some individuals, and the risk of deep-vein thrombosis is increased in women who are obese, hypertensive or smokers. Those individuals who have Factor V Leiden have an increased incidence of deep-vein thrombosis with oral contraceptive use. There is evidence that Factor V Leiden in postmenopausal women on HT is also associated with an increased incidence of venous thrombosis.

Women who have had a prior deep-vein thrombosis, pulmonary emboli or a strong family history of thrombosis should have blood coagulation profiles carried out (Table 11.5). If a woman has a history of well-documented deep-vein thrombosis or pulmonary emboli, then the use of oral estrogens is contraindicated. Transdermal estrogens have less of an effect on blood coagulation factors than oral estrogens, and some evidence suggests that they are less thrombogenic: in a study of 155 women, Scarabin et al. found that oral estrogen was associated with thromboembolism four times more often than was transdermal estrogen (3.5 vs 0.9).

Individuals using HT who develop a deep-vein thrombosis or pulmonary embolus should discontinue the therapy. The usual

TABLE 11.5

Suggested investigations in women with a history of deep-vein thrombosis or pulmonary emboli

Factor	Result associated with increased risk of thrombosis
Fibrinogen	Higher than normal levels
Antithrombin III	Lower than normal levels
Protein C	Lower than normal levels
Protein S	Lower than normal levels
Factor V Leiden	Present

management includes anticoagulants such as heparin or warfarin sodium. Recent publications indicate that anticoagulation therapy should be continued for at least 1 year. Following the use of anticoagulants, aspirin therapy is indicated on an indefinite basis. If the woman is satisfactorily treated with anticoagulants, the concomitant administration of HT does not increase the risk of recurrent thrombosis or emboli.

Recent data suggest that the use of aspirin and/or statin therapy reduces the occurrence of venous thrombosis in women using HT.

Insulin and glucose metabolism. There is no evidence that estrogen or EPT increases the incidence of diabetes. Recent evidence has suggested that there is actually a decrease in the occurrence of carbohydrate intolerance in women using HT.

Breast cancer. There have been many reports of an increase, a decrease and no change in the incidence of breast cancer with estrogen or estrogen plus progestogen replacement therapy. In the WHI study, there was no statistically significant increase in the incidence of breast cancer during the first 5 years of HT among women who had not previously used HT (Figure 11.2).

Women who have used HT for more than 5 years appear to have an increased risk of being diagnosed with breast cancer. There are observational data indicating that this increased risk is greater in women on estrogen plus progestogen compared with estrogen only. One intriguing finding is that, on stopping therapy, women who have used HT for 10 or more years return, within 2 to 5 years, to a risk level similar to where they would be if they had never used HT.

These data support the picture of increasing mitotic activity with HT, causing either growth or a new mutation in the nuclear DNA. This is in contrast to the supposition that estrogen or estrogen plus progestogen is a cause of the neoplasia.

It has been recommended that women stop HT after 5 years of use. Another option is to maintain HT but evaluate women regularly (including with mammography). This approach should be considered for symptomatic women at low risk for breast cancer.

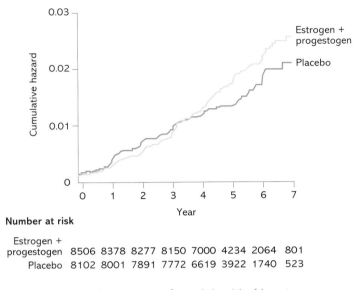

Number at risk

Estrogen + progestogen	8506	8378	8277	8150	7000	4234	2064	801
Placebo	8102	8001	7891	7772	6619	3922	1740	523

Figure 11.2 Kaplan–Meier estimate of cumulative risk of breast cancer among postmenopausal women taking estrogen plus progestogen compared with women taking placebo. Reproduced with permission from the Writing Group for the Women's Health Initiative Investigators. *JAMA* 2002;288:321–33.

Suppressor genes. Each cell contains suppressor genes such as *BRCA1, BRCA2, p16, p18, p21, p23, p27* and *p53*. These suppressor genes are often expressed following a mutation. A small percentage of people inherit chromosomal abnormalities within specific suppressor genes such as *BRCA1* or *BRCA2*, which makes them incapable of correcting oncogenic changes. Women who are positive for mutations in *BRCA1* or *BRCA2* should not use HT unless there is a very strong case for use because symptoms are affecting their quality of life.

The media. From 2002 onwards, several reports from the large prospective randomized WHI trial have been released. These reports have been given wide publicity, with what can only be called 'soundbite' reporting. One or two outcomes from each of the reports are dramatically presented to the public indicating real or potential problems with the use of HT. Breast cancer, although having an increased relative hazard, was not found to be statistically significantly increased in the WHI data (see Figure 11.2). Women who had previously used HT for 5 or more years were shown to have an increased incidence of breast cancer. Similar data have been reported from the Million Women Study in the UK. Again, the issue is one of HT being causal. This is difficult to trace in the medical literature. Epidemiological and randomized controlled trials only show associations and not causality.

It is important to understand that breast cancer occurs in older women; 80% of breast cancers occur in women who have never received HT. This incidence of breast cancer increases linearly with advancing age (Figure 11.3).

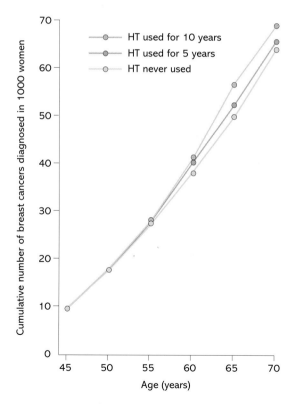

Figure 11.3 Breast cancer is a disease of older women; the risk of being diagnosed with breast cancer increases linearly with age. Data from Collaborative Group on Hormonal Factors in Breast Cancer. *Lancet* 1997;350:1047–59.

The attributable risk or incidence of breast cancer at age 50 is approximately 2 cases per 100 women; if they never use HT, the incidence of breast cancer rises to approximately 4 cases per 100 women at the age of 60. If there is an increase in the relative risk of breast cancer, and let us say that it is 26% as in the WHI results, this translates into an increase in the total number of cases of no more than approximately 0.75 new cases of breast cancer per 100 women who have used HT over a 5-year period. This is an important point, since many women believe the 26% increase in the risk is directly related to themselves and therefore that would mean that they have a 26% increase in the chance of developing breast cancer. This reasoning is obviously fallacious and needs to be brought out specifically in counseling women on their risk related to their age.

Managing issues. Over the past several decades, there has been much controversy among the medical profession and the lay public about the role of hormones and breast cancer. Some of the most frequently asked questions and their answers are discussed in Table 11.6.

TABLE 11.6

Frequently asked questions about hormone therapy (HT) and breast cancer

Do hormones cause breast cancer? Hormones do not cause breast cancer. However, hormones can influence the rate of mitosis and therefore, indirectly, the rate at which oncogenic mutations occur. Estrogen increases mitotic activity in ductal cells and thus has the potential to increase the rate of growth of cells that have already undergone those mutations that ultimately lead to cancer. Progestogens exert their major influence on lobular cells, inducing an initial stimulus to cell division, but eventually leading to differentiation and maturation.

TABLE 11.6

Frequently asked questions about HT and breast cancer (continued)

There is no biological evidence that progestogens actually cause oncogenic mutations, but they do increase mitosis in alveolar cells; see Wren BG. *Climacteric* 2004;7:120–8.

Should women with lumpy/cystic/tender breasts use HT?
Lumps in the breasts are generally fibroadenoma masses caused by fibrous reaction in the fat tissue that surrounds the glands. Fibroadenomas feel fine, granular and gritty to palpation, or like a diffuse rubbery mass. Fibroadenomas are generally smooth, round or oval and do not attach to the skin, underlying tissue or nipple. They are generally tender to compression. There is no more likelihood of these lesions becoming malignant than any other breast tissue. If cancer does occur in the area near the fibroadenoma, it may be more difficult to detect clinically. Women with fibroadenomas should be advised to have regular mammograms and/or ultrasound examinations if indicated. If there is any doubt regarding the etiology of the breast lump, then a fine-needle biopsy should be performed. As stressed earlier, hormones do not induce oncogenic changes in this type of tissue, and continuous combined HT can be given to women with fibroadenomas.

Can women with a family history of breast cancer be given HT? Current evidence indicates that women with a family history of breast cancer fall into two distinct groups. Principally, there are those who have a relative in whom breast cancer occurred at an early age. This group is the smaller, accounting for approximately 5% of women with a family history. These women frequently have the inherited defective *BRCA1* and *BRCA2* genes. They are always at an increased risk of breast cancer from an early age, and are generally advised that HT is not suitable. However, if symptoms are severe then they may be given HT or an alternative such as tibolone.

CONTINUED

TABLE 11.6

Frequently asked questions about HT and breast cancer (continued)

The second group of women are those with a family history of breast cancer in a sibling or mother that developed at a later age. Frequently the breast cancer occurs after the age of 60 in these relatives. This type of breast cancer could be construed as being more likely spontaneous and sporadic rather than as real evidence of a genetic inheritance. In the WHI trial, family history of breast cancer was not found to be a risk factor for developing breast cancer in women taking HT. Other data have also supported this finding, and therefore the family history of breast cancer appears to be only of significance if it is consistent in the family through several generations and/or associated with an early onset of breast cancer (under 45).

Can women who have had breast cancer be given HT?
Women who have had breast cancer are often told by their oncologists never to use HT. This advice is really not based on fact. Much trial evidence has been reassuring, and most studies have shown no increased risk of recurrence or increased mortality associated with HT after treatment for breast cancer, but the Danish HABITS (Hormone Replacement Therapy After Breast Cancer – Is It Safe?) trial was stopped prematurely in 2003 because of a slight increase of recurrence after breast-cancer treatment.

The question is particularly relevant because of the increased severity and incidence of menopausal symptoms in younger women who have undergone either chemotherapy or radiation therapy for the treatment of their breast cancer. This group of women often find that their quality of life is significantly reduced secondary to their therapy and opt to use hormones for management.

Women with early-stage breast cancer have a cure rate approaching 90%. If the cancer has been cured or eliminated, then hormones do not initiate a new cancer. However, if there is a viable cancer cell still present following treatment, then hormones will promote an earlier recurrence and possible earlier death. Individual

TABLE 11.6

Frequently asked questions about HT and breast cancer (continued)

women must be told the risk potential and possibility of recurrence in such cases. Specialist advice for those with severe and distressing menopausal symptoms will allow the woman herself to weigh the evidence and make an informed choice.

A further issue in this group of women is the frequency with which physicians underdiagnose the occurrence of depression. Antidepressant medication should be considered in these women not only to relieve their menopausal symptoms (specifically hot flashes), but also to improve their general mood.

Can estrogens be used with antiestrogens such as tamoxifen? Tamoxifen has been studied in depth and has been found to reduce the recurrence rate of breast cancer by approximately 50%. Tamoxifen itself has a weak estrogenic activity, and it is associated with both an increased risk of thrombosis as well as atypical changes in the endometrium. At present, although the theoretical consideration would be compelling for the use of both tamoxifen and estrogen together, it does not represent an acceptable standard of care.

Endometrial cancer. The different breast cancer risks reported by WHI for women using estrogen alone and estrogen plus progestogen has opened debate on whether women who have a uterus should consider using estrogen without progestogen. It is argued by some that the breast cancer risk difference could justify accepting the small risk of endometrial cancer known to be associated with unopposed estrogen use. Although some women on unopposed estrogen do not bleed, many eventually have troublesome bleeding, and many gynecologists would argue that the combination of endometrial safety and control of bleeding still carries the argument in favor of opposed estrogen, as has been the case for the past 25 years.

Key points – risks of hormone therapy

- Most cancers occur as a result of a sequence of mutations involving promoters and inhibitors in otherwise normal cells.
- Sex hormone therapy is not mutagenic but does increase mitotic activity.
- Oral estrogen may increase the production of thrombogenic proteins from the liver whereas transdermal therapy may reduce this risk.
- Medical research involves results from biological science, clinical application and epidemiological studies. When there is a discrepancy between the results from one discipline to another, it is likely that some of the data are flawed.
- Whilst the most important risks associated with HT are stroke, venous thrombosis and breast cancer, the best randomized clinical trial evidence indicates that the absolute risk from HT is low in women in the early postmenopausal years and increases with increasing age, to be highest in women over 70 years.

Key references

Beral V, Banks E, Reeves G. Evidence from randomised trials on the long-term effects of hormone replacement therapy. *Lancet* 2002;360:942–44.

British Menopause Society. *BMS Council Consensus Statement on Hormone Replacement Therapy* June 2004. www.the-bms.org/consensus.htm

International Menopause Society. Guidelines for hormone treatment of women in the menopausal transition and beyond. Position Statement by the Executive Committee of the International Menopause Society [revised 15 October 2004]. *Climacteric* 2004;7:333–7. www.imsociety.org/PDF/news_IMS_statement_15.10.04.pdf?PHPSESS ID=5c0fdb961379784326119d3c3f cb2c04

North American Menopause Society. Recommendations for estrogen and progestogen use in peri- and postmenopausal women: October 2004 position statement of The North American Menopause Society. *Menopause* 2004;11:589–600. www.menopause.org/edumaterials/ 2004HTreport.pdf

Rees M, Purdie DW, eds. *Management of the Menopause*, 3rd edn. Marlow: BMS Publications, 2002.

Writing Group for the Women's Health Initiative Investigators. Risks and benefits of estrogen plus progestin in healthy menopausal women. *JAMA* 2002;288:321–33.

Thrombosis and embolism

Daly E, Vessey MP, Hawkins MM et al. Risk of venous thromboembolism in users of hormone replacement therapy. *Lancet* 1996;348:977–80.

Grodstein F, Stampfer MJ, Goldhaber SZ et al. Prospective study of exogenous hormones and risk of pulmonary embolism in women. *Lancet* 1996;348:983–7.

Scarabin PY, Oger E, Plu-Bureau G; EStrogen and THromboEmbolism Risk Study Group. Differential association of oral and transdermal oestrogen-replacement therapy with venous thromboembolism risk. *Lancet* 2003;362:428–32.

Cancer

Beresford SAA, Weiss NS, Voigt LF et al. Risk of endometrial cancer in relation to use of estrogen combined with cyclic progestogen therapy in postmenopausal women. *Lancet* 1997;349:458–61.

Clarke CL, Sutherland RL. Progestin regulation of cellular proliferation. *Endocr Rev* 1990;11:266–301.

Col NF, Hirota LK, Orr RK et al. Hormone replacement therapy after breast cancer: a systematic review and quantitative assessment of risk. *J Clin Oncol* 2001;19:2357–63.

Colditz GA, Hankinson SE, Hunter DA et al. The use of estrogens and progestins and the risk of breast cancer in postmenopausal women. *N Engl J Med* 1995;332: 1589–93.

Collaborative Group on Hormonal Factors in Breast Cancer. Breast cancer and hormone replacement therapy: collaborative re-analysis of data from 51 epidemiologic studies of 52 705 women with breast cancer and 108 411 women without breast cancer. *Lancet* 1997;350:1047–59.

Eden JA, Bush TL, Nand S et al. A case control study of combined continuous estrogen–progestin replacement therapy among women with a personal history of breast cancer. *Menopause* 1995;2:67–72.

Grady D, Gebretsadik T, Kerlikowske K et al. Hormone replacement therapy and endometrial cancer risk: a meta-analysis. *Obstet Gynecol* 1995;85:304–13.

Lando JF. Hormone replacement therapy and breast cancer risk in a nationally representative cohort. *Am J Prev Med* 1999;17:176–80.

Musgrove EA, Hui R, Sweeney KJE et al. Cyclins and breast cancer. *J Mammary Gland Biol Neopl* 1996;1:153–62.

Musgrove EA, Lee CSL, Sutherland RL. Progestins both stimulate and inhibit breast cancer cell cycle progression while increasing expression of transforming growth factor a, epidermal growth factor receptor, c-fos and c-myc genes. *Mol Cell Biol* 1991;11:5032–43.

O'Meara ES, Rossing MA, Daling JR et al. Hormone replacement therapy after a diagnosis of breast cancer in relation to recurrence and mortality. *J Natl Cancer Inst* 2001;93:754–62.

Plu-Bureau G, Le MG, Sitruk-Ware R et al. Progestogen use and decreased risk of breast cancer in a cohort study of premenopausal women with benign breast disease. *Br J Cancer* 1994;70:270–7.

Ross RK, Paganini-Hill AA, Wan PC et al. Effect of hormone replacement therapy on breast cancer risk: estrogen versus estrogen plus progestin. *J Natl Cancer Inst* 2000;92:328–32.

Royal College of Obstetricians and Gynaecologists Guideline No. 12. *Pregnancy after Breast Cancer*. London: Royal College of Obstetricians and Gynaecologists, 1997.

Schairer C, Lubin J, Troisi R et al. Menopausal estrogen and estrogen-progestin replacement therapy and breast cancer risk. *JAMA* 2000;283: 485–91.

Sherr CJ, Roberts JM. Inhibitors of mammalian G1 cyclin-dependent kinases. *Genes Dev Rev* 1995;9: 1149–63.

Woodruff JD, Pickar JH. Incidence of endometrial hyperplasia in postmenopausal women taking conjugated estrogens (Premarin) with medroxyprogesterone acetate or conjugated estrogens alone. The Menopause Study Group. *Am J Obstet Gynecol* 1994;170:1213–23.

Wren BG. Do female sex hormones initiate breast cancer? A review of the evidence. *Climacteric* 2004;7: 120–28.

Wren BG, Eden JA. Do progestogens reduce the risk of breast cancer: a review of the evidence. *Menopause* 1996;3:4–12.

Zumoff B. Editorial: The critical role of alcohol consumption in determining the risk of breast cancer with postmenopausal estrogen administration. *J Clin Endocr Metab* 1997;82:1656–8.

HT with estrogen is not suitable for all women for a number of reasons, including a dislike of vaginal bleeding, development of an unacceptable side effect (such as breast tenderness, headache, weight gain) or concern about the risks associated with its use (primarily breast or endometrial cancer, or thrombosis); in some women, estrogen is relatively or absolutely contraindicated. Women avoiding estrogen but with severe or unacceptable menopausal symptoms will seek an alternative, of which there are several, each with its own profile of advantages and disadvantages (see Table 13.1, page 93).

Tibolone belongs to a class of steroid compounds that regulate estrogenic activity in a tissue-selective manner, the selective tissue estrogenic activity regulators (STEARs). The clinical profile of tibolone is different from that of estrogen or estrogen plus progestogen treatments (EPT). It may be used to treat climacteric symptoms and prevent bone loss, but it does not stimulate the endometrium and breast. The main advantages of tibolone over other hormonal therapies are:

- it does not cause endometrial hyperplasia
- it has a low incidence of venous thromboembolism
- it does not increase mammographic density.

Metabolism, kinetics and receptor activation
After oral administration, tibolone is very rapidly metabolized to 3α- and 3β-hydroxytibolone (Figure 12.1). These two compounds are responsible for the estrogenic activity of tibolone. A third metabolite, the Δ^4 isomer, disappears from the circulation as rapidly as tibolone.

Effects of tibolone
Breast. Tibolone and its metabolites do not inhibit aromatase, but sulfatase is profoundly inhibited, so that the conversion of inactive

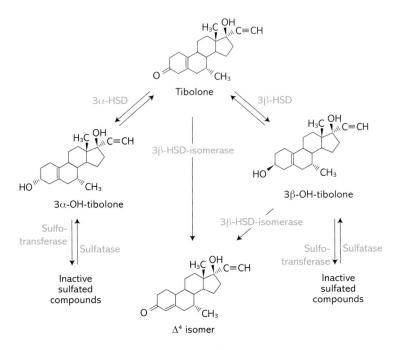

Figure 12.1 The metabolism of tibolone. HSD, hydroxysteroid dehydrogenase.

estrone sulfate to active estrone is reduced. Tibolone not only inhibits proliferation of normal breast epithelial cells but also stimulates apoptosis. In this respect, tibolone behaves differently from estrogens. In clinical studies, tibolone users do not show the increase in mammographic density observed with continuous combined EPT, and experience less breast tenderness.

Endometrium. The progestogenic effects on the endometrium are mediated via tibolone and its Δ^4 isomer. Clinically, there is no difference between the effects of tibolone and continuous combined hormone therapy on endometrial thickness, but the incidence of vaginal bleeding is lower with tibolone. The endometrium remains atrophic in the majority of women treated with tibolone.

Cardiovascular system and lipid profile. The effects of tibolone on plasma lipids are well known. It decreases high-density lipoprotein

> **Key points – tibolone**
>
> - Tibolone is a selective tissue estrogenic activity regulator, with estrogenic and progestogenic metabolites.
> - Tibolone is an effective option for menopausal symptom relief.
> - Tibolone has been shown to preserve bone mass.

(HDL) cholesterol levels, lipoprotein(a) and triglycerides (associated with a reduction in circulating remnants). However, the clinical effect of tibolone on the cardiovascular response is uncertain.

Menopausal symptoms. Randomized, placebo-controlled studies have confirmed that tibolone is highly effective in controlling hot flashes, sweating and other typical postmenopausal symptoms such as fatigue, nervousness, headache and insomnia.

Sexual wellbeing. The tissue-selective effect of tibolone on the lower urogenital tract leads to relief of urogenital symptoms and restores a healthy vaginal environment.

Tibolone has a positive effect on sexual wellbeing, with a significantly increased vaginal blood flow, greater sexual desire, vaginal lubrication and frequency of arousability and sexual fantasies. In addition to its estrogenic effects, tibolone also induces changes in androgen status that may contribute towards its greater effect on sexual wellbeing than that seen with EPT.

Bone mineral density. Tibolone inhibits markers of bone resorption and bone formation, preventing bone loss and increasing bone mineral density in postmenopausal women. Clinical studies have confirmed that it exerts effects on the skeleton similar to those shown by estrogen regimens. Studies demonstrating the effect of tibolone on fracture rates are awaited.

Key references

Bruce D, Robinson J, Rymer J. Long-term effects of tibolone on the endometrium as assessed by bleeding episodes, transvaginal scan and endometrial biopsy. *Climacteric* 2004;7:261–6.

de Gooyer ME, Deckers GH, Schoonen WG et al. Receptor profiling and endocrine interactions of tibolone. *Steroids* 2003;68:21–30.

Devogelaer JP. A review of the effects of tibolone on the skeleton. *Expert Opin Pharmacother* 2004;5:941–9.

Huber J, Palacios S, Berglund L et al. Effects of tibolone and continuous combined hormone replacement therapy on bleeding rates, quality of life and tolerability in postmenopausal women. *BJOG* 2002;109:886–93.

Kenemans P, Speroff L. Tibolone: Clinical recommendations and practical guidelines. A report of the International Tibolone Consensus Group. *Maturitas* 2005;51:21–8.

Kloosterboer HJ. Tissue-selective effects of tibolone on the breast. *Maturitas* 2004;49:S5–S15.

Kloosterboer HJ. Tissue-selectivity: the mechanism of action of tibolone. *Maturitas* 2004;48(suppl 1):S30–S40.

Kovalevsky G. Female sexual dysfunction and use of hormone therapy in postmenopausal women. *Semin Reprod Med* 2005;23:180–7.

Landgren MB, Helmond FA, Engelen S. Tibolone relieves climacteric symptoms in highly symptomatic women with at least seven hot flushes and sweats per day. *Maturitas* 2005;50:222–30.

Modelska K, Cummings S. Tibolone for postmenopausal women: systematic review of randomized trials. *J Clin Endocrinol Metab* 2002;87:16–23.

Valdivia I, Campodonico I, Tapia A et al. Effects of tibolone and continuous combined hormone therapy on mammographic breast density and breast histochemical markers in postmenopausal women. *Fertil Steril* 2004;81:617–23.

von Schoultz B. The effects of tibolone and oestrogen-based HT on breast cell proliferation and mammographic density. *Maturitas* 2004;49:S16–S21.

Although some women unhappy with the side effects or possible consequences of HT may simply discontinue treatment, others may explore therapies that provide some of the benefits of HT with fewer risks. Each alternative has its own profile of advantages and disadvantages (Table 13.1).

Selective estrogen-receptor modulators

Selective estrogen-receptor modulators (SERMs) were originally used in the management of breast cancer and ovulation induction because of their antiestrogenic effects. Since then, SERMs have also been shown to exert estrogenic effects. The newer generations are in development, and raloxifene is now available in many countries.

Raloxifene has been shown to bind to estrogen receptors and subsequently induce expression of estrogen-responsive genes in some, but not all, estrogen-sensitive tissues. Raloxifene and estrogens, acting via the same receptor, can induce different receptor conformations that result in different biological responses. In

TABLE 13.1

Hormone therapy is not the only option for postmenopausal symptoms

Symptom/system	Alternative agents
Vasomotor	Tibolone, phytoestrogens, clonidine
Psychological	Tibolone, phytoestrogens
Urogenital atrophy	Tibolone, phytoestrogens
Osteoporosis	Tibolone, bisphosphonates, calcitonin, SERMs, phytoestrogens, calcium ± vitamin D
Cardiovascular system	Tibolone, SERMs, phytoestrogens

SERMs, selective estrogen-receptor modulators.

addition, some SERMs and estrogens act on α- and β-receptors to produce different responses in different tissues.

Raloxifene does not appear to stimulate the postmenopausal uterus or breast significantly. Consequently, its side-effect profile is substantially improved compared with HT. Indeed, in the Multiple Outcomes of Raloxifene Evaluation (MORE) randomized controlled trial for the treatment of osteoporosis, there were significantly fewer new breast-cancer diagnoses for raloxifene than for placebo. Thus the risk of breast cancer may be reduced in women using raloxifene. There does, however, appear to be a small increase in the risk of venous thrombosis, similar to that with HT.

Treatment with raloxifene has a number of benefits; there is evidence that it significantly preserves bone and reduces vertebral fractures in postmenopausal women compared with placebo. Further data suggest that raloxifene may protect the cardiovascular system, but the available evidence is less extensive than it is for estrogen.

Raloxifene does not relieve vasomotor symptoms, and may even increase flashes in some women. In clinical trials, less than 20% of women receiving the drug were affected by flashes. The effect on urogenital tissues is variable, with some women experiencing considerable improvement while others remain unaffected. The effect on brain function is not yet clear.

Overall, raloxifene and possibly other SERMs in development offer a degree of skeletal, and possibly cardiovascular, protection without the risks of cancer and vaginal bleeding that are associated with HT. There is evidence that the risk of breast cancer may be reduced in women using raloxifene. It does not appear to offer relief from acute menopausal symptoms. Many women might find raloxifene an acceptable alternative if they were able to avoid the flashes.

Phytoestrogens

Phytoestrogens may be estrogenic or antiestrogenic in their action, depending on the level of estradiol available and other factors. The most important members of this family of substances and their sources are shown in Table 13.2.

TABLE 13.2

Major phytoestrogens

Phytoestrogen	Principal agents	Sources
Isoflavones	Genistein Daidzein Equol	Legumes, particularly soy and soy products
Lignans	Enterodiol Enterolactone	Grains, particularly linseed Cereals

Interest in phytoestrogens has been stimulated by the different disease profiles observed in Asian populations, such as the Japanese, who have phytoestrogen-rich diets. These differences include lower incidences of menopausal flashes, breast and prostate cancers, and cardiovascular disease. Such soy-rich diets may contain levels of phytoestrogens 10- to 20-fold higher than those in a typical Western diet. In Japanese women, the level of intake of isoflavones is such that, despite the relatively low estrogenic potency of isoflavones, the circulating level can be up to a thousand times higher than that of estradiol. Clinical trials are under way to investigate the use of phytoestrogens in the management of menopausal symptoms. Administration as dietary supplements or purified extracts from dietary sources is being investigated.

To date, the available evidence suggests that phytoestrogens have some action in the prevention of menopausal flashes, but less on urogenital atrophy. There is no clinical evidence concerning cardiovascular outcomes, but mechanistic studies, particularly in monkeys, suggest that the processes of atheroma formation are less marked with a soy-rich diet. It is likely that, over the next 5–10 years, the significance of phytoestrogens will be established, and more products containing phytoestrogens will be available.

Many women have great faith in herbal products as a substitute for natural estrogen. It is best to consider phytoestrogens as a useful addition to, rather than a substitute for, HT.

Key points – alternatives to hormone therapy

- Raloxifene does not reduce menopausal symptoms, but preserves bone mass and has been shown to reduce spinal fracture rates. There is a significant reduction in rates of breast cancer in postmenopausal women not selected for their breast-cancer risk.
- Phytoestrogen therapies have been proposed for menopausal symptom relief.
- There is an inadequate evidence base to justify the use of complementary therapies in menopausal symptom relief.
- Regular exercise is associated with a range of health benefits.

Complementary medicine

Many women who use complementary approaches are satisfied with the results, but there is a lack of clinical trial evidence concerning their effect on menopausal symptoms. This lack of evidence is an important consideration as the treatment of menopausal symptoms, particularly hot flashes, is associated with a significant placebo response. For flashes, the placebo effect is approximately 30%. Complementary therapies that can be explored include homeopathy, acupuncture, reflexology and aromatherapy.

Exercise

Regular exercise has a role to play in the prevention of cardiovascular disease, and regular weight-bearing exercise can help to reduce the risk of osteoporosis. Exercise should be a continuing activity throughout an individual's life to have an effect on long-term health. It has also been suggested that exercise has a positive influence on a woman's sense of well-being, and this in turn may have a positive effect on flashes.

Key references

Bassey EJ. Exercise for prevention of osteoporotic fracture. *Age Ageing* 2001;30(suppl 4):29–31.

Cummings SR, Eckert S, Krueger KA et al. The effect of raloxifene on risk of breast cancer in postmenopausal women: results from the MORE randomized trial. Multiple Outcomes of Raloxifene Evaluation. *JAMA* 1999;281:2189–97.

Delmas PD, Ensrud KE, Adachi JD et al. Multiple Outcomes of Raloxifene Evaluation Investigators. Efficacy of raloxifene on vertebral fracture risk reduction in postmenopausal women with osteoporosis: four-year results from a randomized clinical trial. *J Clin Endocrinol Metab* 2002;87:3609–17.

Ettinger B, Black DM, Mitlak BH et al. Reduction of vertebral fracture risk in postmenopausal women with osteoporosis treated with raloxifene: results from a 3-year randomized clinical trial. Multiple Outcomes of Raloxifene Evaluation (MORE) Investigators. *JAMA* 1999;282: 637–45.

Glazier MG, Bowman MA. A review of the evidence for the use of phytoestrogens as a replacement for traditional estrogen replacement therapy. *Arch Intern Med* 2001;161:1161–72.

Useful resources

American Menopause Foundation
National Headquarters
350 Fifth Avenue, Suite 2822
New York, NY 10118
www.americanmenopause.org

Australasian Menopause Society
PO Box 1228
Buderim, QLD 4556
Tel: +61 7 5456 2660
Fax: +61 7 5456 2661
ams@netlink.com.au
www.menopause.org.au

British Menopause Society
4–6 Eton Place
Marlow, Bucks SL7 2QA
Tel: +44 (0)1628 890199
Fax: +44 (0)1628 474042
www.the-bms.org.uk

Daisy Network (UK) (for women
suffering premature menopause)
PO Box 183
Rossendale BB4 6WZ
www.daisynetwork.org.uk

Early Menopause Australia Support
Group
www.jeanhailes.org.au/issues/mp_e
arly_ema.htm

European Menopause and
Andropause Society
emas.obgyn.net

International Menopause Society
Jean Wright, IMS Executive
Director
PO Box 687, Wray
Lancaster LA2 8WY
Tel: +44 (0)15242 21190
Fax: +44 (0)15242 22596
jwright.ims@btopenworld.com
www.imsociety.org

National Osteoporosis Foundation
(USA)
1232 22nd Street N.W.
Washington, DC 20037-1292
Tel: +1 202 223 2226
www.nof.org

National Osteoporosis Society (UK)
Camerton
Bath BA2 0PJ
Tel: +44 (0)1761 471771 (for
general enquiries)
Helpline: 0845 4500230 (for
medical queries)
Fax: +44 (0)1761 471104
info@nos.org.uk
www.nos.org.uk

North American Menopause Society

PO Box 94527

Cleveland, OH 44101

Tel: + 1440 442 7550

Fax: +1 440 442 2660

info@menopause.org

www.menopause.org

Osteoporosis Society of Canada

33 Laird Drive, Toronto

Ontario M4G 3S9

Tel: +1 416 696 2663

Toll-free (English): 800 463 6842

(in Canada only)

Toll-free (French): 800 977 1778

(in Canada only)

Fax: +1 416 696 2673

osc@osteoporosis.ca

www.osteoporosis.ca

Women's Health Concern (UK)

PO Box 2126, Marlow

Bucks SL7 2RY

Tel: +44 (0)1628 488065

Fax: +44 (0)1628 474042

Helpline: 0845 123 2319

counselling@womens-health-
concern.org

www.womens-health-concern.org

Books for patients

Wren, BG. *Understanding the
Menopause and Hormonal
Therapy.* 2nd edn. Sydney,
McGraw–Hill, 2004.

Appendix

Generic and proprietary names of estrogens

Proprietary name (USA)	Proprietary name (UK)	Proprietary name (Australia)
Conjugated estrogens with progestogen		
Premphase (t)	Premique (t)	Premia (t)
Prempro (t)	Prempak-C (t)	Provelle (t)
		Menoprem (t)
Estradiol with progestogen		
Activella (t)	Adgyn Combi (t)	Climen (t)
Climara Pro (p)	Climagest (t)	Climen 28 (t)
CombiPatch (p)	Climesse (t)	Divina (t)
FemHRT (t)	Cyclo-Progynova (t)	Estracombi
Ortho-Prefest (t)	Elleste-Duet (t)	Femoston (t)
	Estracombi (t, p)	Estalis 50/140 (p)
	Estrapak 50 (t, p)	Estalis 50/250 (p)
	Evorel (p ± t)	Kliogest (t)
	Femapak (t, p)	Kliovance (t)
	Femoston (t)	
	FemSeven Conti (p)	
	FemSeven Sequi (t, p)	
	Indivina (t)	
	Kliofem (t)	
	Kliovance (t)	
	Nuvelle (t)	
	Tridestra (t)	
	Trisequens (t)	

Proprietary name (USA)	Proprietary name (UK)	Proprietary name (Australia)
Conjugated estrogens only		
Cenestin (t)	Premarin (t)	Premarin (t)
Premarin (t)		Primogyn Depot (inj)
Esterified estrogens		
MenEst (t)		
Estradiol only		
Alora (p)	Adgyn Estro (t)	Aerodiol (n)
Climara (p)	Aerodiol (n)	Climara (p)
Esclim (p)	Climaval (t)	Dermestril (p)
Estrace (t)	Dermestril (p)	Estraderm (p)
Estraderm (p)	Dermestril-Septem (p)	Estraderm MX (p)
Estrasorb (c)	Elleste-Solo (p)	Estradiol implants (i)
Estrogel (g)	Elleste-Solo MX (p)	Estrofem (t)
FemPatch (p)	Estraderm MX (p)	Femtran (p)
FemRing (r)	Estraderm TTS (p)	Menorest (p)
Gynodiol (t)	Estradiol implants (i)	Progynova (t)
Vagifem (v)	Evorel (p)	Sandrena (g)
Vivelle (p)	Fematrix (p)	Zumenon (t)
	FemSeven (p)	
	Menorest (p)	
	Menoring 50 (r)	
	Oestrogel (g)	
	Progynova (t)	
	Progynova TS (p)	
	Sandrena (g)	
	Vagifem (v)	
	Zumenon (t)	

Proprietary name (USA)	Proprietary name (UK)	Proprietary name (Australia)
Estradiol, estriol and estrone only		
Tri-Est* (c, g)	Hormonin (t)	
Estriol only		
	Ovestin (t)	Ovestin (t)
Estropipate only		
Ogen (t)	Harmogen (t)	Genoral (t)
Ortho-Est (t)		Ogen (t)
Estrogen and testosterone		
Estratest (t)		

*This and other formulations are available from pharmacists, who can make up estrogen-containing creams, gels or capsules to prescription.
c, cream; g, gel; i, implant; inj, injection; n, nasal spray; p, patch; r, vaginal ring; t, tablet; v, vaginal tablet.

Index

acne 43, 57–8
age
  breast cancer risk 81–2
  HT risks 68–9, 75–6, 77
  menopause and related symptoms 10, 22, 26, 29
alendronate 40
Alzheimer's disease 29, 31, 42
androgens
  androgenic progestogens 57
  testosterone 35–6, 43
anticoagulants 79
aspirin 79
atherosclerosis 30, 63–4, 75–6
Australia 18, 40

β-amyloid 31
bisphosphonates 39–40
bladder see urogenital system
bloating 55–6
blood pressure 65, 77
bone loss see osteoporosis
bowel cancer 74
BRCA1/2 mutations 80, 83
breakthrough bleeding 47, 60–1, 85
breast
  cancer 67, 71, 74, 79–85, 94
  effect of steroids 56–7, 65–7, 82, 89–90
  pain 56–7

calcitonin 40
calcium 41
cancer
  bowel 74
  breast 67, 71, 74, 79–85, 94
  endometrium 47, 52, 60, 74, 85

cardiovascular system
  alternatives to estrogen 90–1, 93, 94, 95, 96
  benefits of estrogen 63–5, 75–6
  risks of HT 49, 66, 68, 72, 75–9
CEE (conjugated equine estrogen) 48
cerebrovascular accidents 30, 71, 74, 76–7
cholesterol 10, 48, 49, 64, 66, 90–1
climacteric 10
clinical trials
  Collaborative Group on Hormones and Cancer 74
  HABITS 84
  HERS 72, 75
  MORE 94
  Nurses Health Study 73
  WHI see Women's Health Initiative
clonidine 38
coagulation 64–5, 66, 77–9
cognitive function 31–2, 42
Collaborative Group on Hormones and Cancer 74
Colles' fractures 22
complementary medicine 96
conjugated equine estrogen (CEE) 48
counseling 37, 47, 82–5
creams 50, 53
curettage 60, 61
cyproterone acetate 58

decision-making ability 30
deep-vein thrombosis see thrombosis
dementia 29, 30, 31, 42
densitometry of bone 19–21
depression 32, 85
dermal patches 49–50, 78

diabetes 79
diet 41, 94–5
DXA (dual-energy X-ray densitometry) 19–21
dydrogesterone 57, 58
dyspareunia 24, 26, 35
dysuria 26

edema 56
embarrassment 25
embolism, pulmonary 77–9
endometrium
  bleeding 46, 47, 60–2, 85
  cancer 47, 52, 60, 74, 85
  effect of tibolone 90
  hyperplasia 47, 50, 52, 60
endothelial-derived relaxing factor (EDRF) 65
endothelium 65, 66
EPT (estrogen plus progestogen) regimes
  clinical trials 63, 71–2, 74, 77, 79
  endometrial bleeding 46, 47, 60, 61
  side effects 57, 58
  types of 11–12, 46–7, 52
esophagus 40
estradiol 48
  see also estrogens
Estring 51
estrogen receptors 31, 94
estrogens
  deficiency 11, 13, 18–19, 29–31, 35, 66
  delivery systems 48–52
  effect on breast tissue 56, 65–7, 82
  function 8–9, 10, 63–5
  metabolism 48
  therapy see hormone therapy
etidronate 40
exercise 96

Factor V Leiden 65, 78
FAI (free androgen index)
43
fibroadenomas 83
flashes (flushes) *see* hot
flashes
formication 15
fracture risk *see*
osteoporosis
FSH (follicle-stimulating
hormone) 7

gallbladder 55
gastrointestinal tract
bowel cancer risk 74
side effects 40, 48, 55–6
gels 50
glucose metabolism 31, 79

HABITS trial 84
HDL cholesterol 49, 66,
90–1
headaches 49, 58
heart
coronary heart disease
71, 72, 76
ventricular function 65,
66
heel ultrasound 21
hemostasis 64–5, 66,
77–9
HERS (Heart and
Estrogen/Progestin
Replacement Study) 72, 75
hip fractures 22–3, 39
hormone therapy (HT)
alternatives to 93–6
clinical trials 39, 42, 63,
67–74, 76–7, 79
effect on symptoms 38,
39, 41, 42, 43, 74
endometrial bleeding 46,
47, 60–2
estrogen plus
progestogen *see* EPT
regimes
estrogen-only regimes
11, 12, 60–1, 70–1, 74
key points 44, 54, 59,
62, 86
pre-prescription checks
37
preparation types
11–12, 46–54

hormone therapy *continued*
risks *see* risks of HT
side effects 47, 49, 53,
55–9
tibolone 67, 89–91
hot flashes 13–17
alternatives to estrogens
38, 91, 93, 94, 95, 96
HT 38, 51–2
hypertension 66, 77
hysterectomy 12, 39

implants 51–2
incontinence 26, 27, 42
inhibin 7
insomnia 29

Japan 95

Lactobacillus 24
LDL cholesterol 48, 49,
64, 66
levonorgestrel 57
libido, loss of 34–6, 43,
91
lipids *see* cholesterol
liver metabolism 48

mastalgia 56–7
memory loss 31–2, 42
menopause, definition
9–10
menorrhagia 61
menstrual cycles 7–10,
37
migraines 49, 58
MORE (Multiple
Outcomes of Raloxifene
Evaluation) 94

neurological symptoms
29–32, 34, 42, 91, 93
neurotransmitters 13, 31
night sweats 15, 29
nitric oxide 65
norethisterone 57
Nurses Health Study 73

oophorectomy 16–17,
38
oral HT 48–9, 52–3, 78
osteoporosis 18–23
treatment 38–41, 74,
91, 94, 96
ovarian function 7–10, 37

parathyroid hormone 41
perimenopause 7–9, 13, 37
phytoestrogens 94–5
piperazine estrone sulfate
48
postmenopause
hormone levels 9
HT 47, 57, 58, 68–72, 76
progestogens
clinical trials 71–2
effect on breast tissue
56, 57, 65, 82–3
endometrial bleeding 60,
61
in HT 11–12, 38, 46–7,
51, 52–3
side effects 55–6, 57–9
psychological symptoms
29–32, 34, 42, 91, 93
pulmonary embolism
77–9

raloxifene 39, 67, 93–4
risedronate 40
risks of HT
cancer (breast) 71, 74,
79–85
cancer (other) 47, 60,
74, 85
cardiovascular 66, 68,
72, 75–9
dementia 29
diabetes 79
key points 86
patient perception of 63,
69, 80–5
WHI results 39, 42, 68,
74, 76–7, 79
see also side effects of
HT

selective estrogen-receptor
modulators (SERMs) 39,
67, 93–4
selective serotonin-
reuptake inhibitors
(SSRI) 43, 52
serotonin agonists 38
sexuality 24, 26, 34–6,
43, 91
side effects of HT 47, 49,
53, 55–9
see also risks of HT

skin
  administration route of
  HT 49–50, 53, 78
  side effects of HT 43,
  57–8
spinal fractures 21–2, 39,
  94
statins 79
stroke 71, 74, 76–7
sweating
  night sweats 15, 29
  use of SSRIs 52
sympathetic nervous
  system 15

T scores 19
tamoxifen 67, 85
temperature regulation
  13–15, 51–2
testosterone 35–6, 43
thrombosis
  HT-related risk 49, 68,
  76, 77–9, 94
  non-HT risk factors 30,
  64–5

tibolone 67, 89–91
transdermal delivery
  systems 49–50, 53, 78

UK 18, 26, 40
ultrasound 21, 60, 61
urinary tract infections 27
urogenital system
  symptoms 24–7, 35
  treatment 41–2, 91, 93
USA 18, 40
uterus *see* endometrium

Vagifem 51
vagina
  symptoms 24, 25, 26,
  27, 35
  treatment 41–2, 50–1,
  91
vasomotor function
  effect of estrogen 13, 65
  symptoms 13–17
  treatment 38, 51–2, 91,
  93, 94, 95, 96
venlafaxine 38

vertebral fractures 21–2,
  39, 94
vitamin D 41

withdrawal bleeding 46,
  47, 60–2
Women's Health Initiative
  (WHI) trial
  cancer risk 74, 79
  cardiovascular risk 69,
  74, 76–7
  dementia risk 42
  fracture risk 39, 74
  study design 63, 67–71
  wrist fractures 22

Z scores 19

What the reviewers say:

concise and well written and accompanied by numerous excellent color illustrations... an excellent little book! Score: 100 - 5 Stars

On *Fast Facts – Sexual Dysfunction* in *Doody's Health Sciences Review*, 2004

it really demystifies the treatments behind this psychiatric disorder

On *Fast Facts – Bipolar Disorders* in *Doody's Health Sciences Review*, 2004

a timely and accessible book... a worthwhile and handy tool for medical students

On *Fast Facts – Dyspepsia*, in *Digestive and Liver Disease* 36, 2004

provides a lot of information in a concise and easily accessible format... a practical guide to managing most lower respiratory tract infections

On *Fast Facts – Respiratory Tract Infection*, in *Respiratory Care* 49(1), 2004

an invaluable guide to the latest thinking

On *Fast Facts – Irritable Bowel Syndrome*, in *Update*, 4 September 2003

a rapid guide to understanding dementia... value for money and I would definitely recommend it

On *Fast Facts – Dementia*, in *South African Medical Journal* 93(10), 2003

excellent coverage of symptoms and diagnosis

On *Fast Facts – Dyspepsia*, in *Update*, 19 June, 2003

will likely be read cover to cover in just one or
two sittings by all who are fortunate enough
to obtain a copy

On *Fast Facts – Benign Prostatic Hyperplasia*, 4th edn, in *Doody's Health Sciences Review*, Dec 2002

explains the important facts and demonstrates
the levels of "good practice" that can be achieved

On *Fast Facts – Minor Surgery*,
in *Journal of the Royal Society for the Promotion of Health* 122(3), 2002

a splendid publication

On *Fast Facts – Sexually Transmitted Infections*, in *Journal of Antimicrobial Chemotherapy* 49, 2002

I would highly recommend it
without reservation... 5 stars!

On *Fast Facts – Psychiatry Highlights 2001–02*,
in *Doody's Health Sciences Review*, Sept 2002

I enthusiastically recommend this
stimulating, short book which should
be required reading for all clinicians

On *Fast Facts – Irritable Bowel Syndrome*, in *Gastroenterology* 120(6), 2001

***** outstanding

On *Fast Facts – HIV in Obstetrics and Gynecology*, in *Journal of Pelvic Surgery*, 2001

a gem for family physicians because of its ease
of use and the sophisticated, concise treatment

On *Fast Facts – Epilepsy*, in *American Family Physician* 64(5), 2001

www.fastfacts.com

FAST FACTS

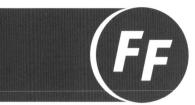

An outstandingly successful independent medical handbook series

Over one million copies sold

- Written by world experts
- Concise and practical
- Up to date
- Designed for ease of reading and reference
- Copiously illustrated with useful photographs, diagrams and charts

Our aim for *Fast Facts* is to be **the world's most respected medical handbook series**. Feedback on how to make titles even more useful is always welcome (feedback@fastfacts.com).

Fast Facts titles include

Acne

Allergic Rhinitis

Asthma

Benign Gynecological Disease (second edition)

Benign Prostatic Hyperplasia (fifth edition)

Bipolar Disorder

Bladder Cancer

Bleeding Disorders

Brain Tumors

Breast Cancer (third edition)

Celiac Disease

Chronic Obstructive Pulmonary Disease

Colorectal Cancer (second edition)

Contraception (second edition)

Dementia

Depression (second edition)

Disorders of the Hair and Scalp

Dyspepsia (second edition)

Eczema and Contact Dermatitis

Endometriosis (second edition)

Epilepsy (second edition)

Erectile Dysfunction (third edition)

Gynecological Oncology

Headaches (second edition)

Hyperlipidemia (third edition)

Hypertension (second edition)

Infant Nutrition

Inflammatory Bowel Disease

Irritable Bowel Syndrome (second edition)

Minor Surgery

Multiple Sclerosis

Osteoporosis (fourth edition)

Parkinson's Disease

Prostate Cancer (fourth edition)

Psoriasis (second edition)

Respiratory Tract Infection (second edition)

Rheumatoid Arthritis

Schizophrenia (second edition)

Sexual Dysfunction

Sexually Transmitted Infections

Smoking Cessation

Soft Tissue Rheumatology

Superficial Fungal Infections

Travel Medicine

Urinary Continence (second edition)

Urinary Stones

Orders

To order via the website, or to find regional distributors, please go to
www.fastfacts.com

For telephone orders, please call +44 (0)1752 202301 (Europe) or
419 281 1802 (North America)